Handbook of Emergency Psychi

Handbook of Emergency Psychiatry

Tom M. Brown
BSc, MPhil, MRCP (UK), MRCPsych
Senior Registrar in Psychiatry
Royal Edinburgh Hospital

Allan I. F. Scott
BSc, MPhil, MRCPsych
Lecturer in Psychiatry
University of Edinburgh

With
Ian M. Pullen
MRCPsych
Consultant Psychiatrist
Royal Edinburgh Hospital
Honorary Senior Lecturer
University of Edinburgh

CHURCHILL LIVINGSTONE
EDINBURGH LONDON MELBOURNE AND NEW YORK 1990

CHURCHILL LIVINGSTONE
Medical Division of Longman Group UK Limited

Distributed in the United States of America by Churchill
Livingstone Inc., 1560 Broadway, New York, N.Y. 10036,
and by associated companies, branches and representatives
throughout the world.

© Longman Group UK Limited 1990

First published 1990

ISBN 0-443-03983-6

British Library Cataloguing in Publication Data
Brown, Tom M.
   Handbook of emergency psychiatry
   1. Medicine. Psychiatry
   I. Title   II. Scott, Allan I. F.   III. Pullen, Ian M.
   616.89

Library of Congress Cataloging-in-Publication Data
Brown, Tom M.
   Handbook of emergency psychiatry/Tom M. Brown, Allan I. F. Scott;
with Ian M. Pullen.
      p.   cm.
   Includes bibliographical references.
      1. Psychiatric emergencies — Handbooks, manuals, etc.   I. Scott,
Allan I. F.   II. Pullen, Ian M.   III. Title.
      [DNLM: 1. Mental Health Services.   WM 401 B881h]
   RC480.6.B76   1990
   616.89′025 — dc20
   DNLM/DLC   89-22106
   for Library of Congress   CIP

Produced by Longman Singapore Publishers (Pte) Ltd.
Printed in Singapore.

Introduction

We decided to write this book while working on the development of a daytime emergency service at the Royal Edinburgh Hospital. In our supervision sessions with junior psychiatric staff, we soon became aware there was little appropriate reading we could recommend to them. Much supervision time was taken up sharing our experiences and discussing what we had learned from difficult cases. Since then more has been written about emergency psychiatry, but to our minds what is available is still too much like textbook psychiatry and fails to tackle many of the practical difficulties that arise. Likewise we have failed to find reading matter that would convey to the doctor new to psychiatry the kinds of common emergencies they will encounter. We hope this book is practical and problem orientated (rather than illness orientated), and will forewarn and guide those without much experience.

This is certainly not a textbook of psychiatry. We assume the readers will have some basic knowledge of psychiatry. Our emphasis is on common clinical problems and their immediate management. Much of this is based on our own experience, and thus not all psychiatrists will agree with everything we write. We have made a conscious decision to be directive in our advice because we feel one of the common difficulties in emergency psychiatry is the worry engendered in the doctor. It can be a lonely experience to take important decisions on your own in the middle of the night. We hope our practical guidelines will bolster confidence in such settings.

For simplicity all patients and doctors are referred to as 'he', although many patients and doctors are female.

We would like to thank the following colleagues for helpful

comment: Dr D. Chiswick, Dr C. P. Freeman, Dr J. Greenwood, Dr A. Jacques, Dr. J. B. Loudon, Dr. G. Masterton, Dr B. Ritson and Dr. P. Semple. We thank Patricia Rose and Marjory Dodd for the preparation of the manuscript.

How to use this book

The principles of assessment and management in emergency psychiatry are covered in Chapters 1–5 and we recommend that everyone should read these chapters first. Subsequent chapters deal with problems that may occur in many different settings, e.g. threats of self-harm, or deal with specific settings, e.g. common problems in casualty departments. All these subsequent chapters make frequent cross-references to the basic principles covered in the first five chapters. This means the chapters are not over-long, and could easily be read before assessing a patient with a particular problem, or being called to a particular setting. Chapter 17 deals specifically with non-medical crisis intervention. No trainee psychiatrist should be without support and supervision in emergency practice, and Chapter 18 is devoted to this. Illustrative case histories of common presenting problems, principles of assessment and management, and some pitfalls are given in Appendix 2. These are numbered and reference is made to these throughout the text. Factual material such as mental health legislation and drug side-effects are also covered in the appendices.

Practice points
These are practical guidelines of major importance which can never be ignored. Several of these occur in each chapter and are denoted by special typography.

This is a practical guide which may be helpful in the middle of the night, but not so appropriate in preparing your differential diagnosis for the professor's ward round. Our aim is to cover the commonplace, not to be exhaustive (or exhausting).

Contents

1. Emergency telephone referrals

AIM

Gather essential information and decide initial response.

INTRODUCTION

Despite the growth of 'walk-in' clinics, many emergency referrals are made by general practitioners (GPs) or other agencies who will telephone to discuss the patient. Remember they may have valuable information that will help you understand the patient, his problem and the supports available.

PRACTICE POINT

At this stage you have control over where and when the patient is seen.

ESSENTIAL INFORMATION ABOUT ANY REFERRAL

Referrer

— Name of person telephoning.
— Organization.
— Contact telephone number.

Patient

— Patient's full name.
— Date of birth.
— Address.

Problem

— Patient's problem, duration and treatment so far.

— Referrer's request, e.g. information, assessment or telephone advice.
— Any specific question, e.g. assessment of suicide risk.

Logistics

— Degree of urgency.
— Where is patient now.
— Legal status, i.e. sectioned or informal.

Previous contact and expectations

— Previous contact with psychiatry.
— Previous contact with this service:
  - If so, roughly when?
  - From what address?
  - Has name changed since then?
  - Record number
— Referrer's expectations, e.g. domiciliary visit, hospital admission.
— GP's name, address and telephone number

PRACTICE POINT
If in doubt give yourself time to think. Say that you will telephone back after consulting the case notes or a colleague.

IMMEDIATE DECISIONS

— Is this the correct service for patient's address or age? Many services now operate a catchment area policy, and elderly patients or the young may have separate services.
— Are you competent to give advice about management over the telephone or should you refer the call to a senior colleague?
— Should the request be passed on to someone else? This will depend on local provision for:
  - Domiciliary visit
  - Assessment of person in police custody
  - Urgent outpatient appointment
— Are you clear about what the referrer is worried, and what he is asking of you?

CONFIDENTIALITY

PRACTICE POINT
Never give information over the telephone unless you know to whom you are talking, and that the caller is entitled to have such information.

Do you know who is calling?

If you do not know and recognize the voice of the person telephoning, how can you be sure he is who he says he is? Patients sometimes masquerade as doctors, social workers or some other person in order to check upon the information they have been given. More sinisterly, the person purporting to be a doctor may be trying to gather information to use against the patient, e.g. in divorce proceedings. Do not give information to a third party without the express consent of the patient.

Divulging personal or medical information

— You may only give privileged medical information to another doctor, and that doctor must have clinical responsibility for the patient, e.g. a casualty officer or a deputizing service GP.
— In an emergency limited information may be given to other professionals where it is essential to the health or safety of a patient, e.g. confirming to the police that a person in custody has a psychiatric history and merits psychiatric assessment.
— Before giving any information take the caller's name, telephone number, organization, profession and the need for the information.
— Ask the switchboard telephonist to check the telephone number of the organization.
— If it is correct, telephone back and ask for the person by name.
— If it is not correct, you may wish to telephone the organization and enquire whether such a person is employed by them and obtain a contact telephone number.
— If in any doubt do not disclose any information. Inform a senior colleague of your concern.

TELEPHONE CALLS FROM PATIENTS OR RELATIVES

Hospital psychiatric services vary in the extent to which such telephone calls or self-referrals are tolerated or encouraged. Callers may seek to:

— Enquire about psychiatric services.
— Obtain support.
— Inform someone of distress or threatened harm.

Enquiries about the psychiatric service

Unless you work in a walk-in emergency clinic or a specialist outpatient service that accepts self-referrals, you should:

— Stress the role of the GP as the source of primary advice:
  • GP will assess the patient's need for psychiatric referral
  • GP will judge the urgency of the referral

Support

Although it can be helpful just to listen to patients in distress, the following points should be borne in mind:

— Is it the role of the duty psychiatrist?
— Should callers be informed about voluntary organizations that carry out such work, e.g. Samaritans?
— Does such support increase dependence on the hospital?
— Ought these problems to be discussed more appropriately with the GP?
— Ought these problems to be discussed with the patient's therapist or key worker — if already attending for treatment?

Patients threatening harm

Callers may say they have taken, or are about to take, an overdose or harm themselves. This puts the duty psychiatrist in an awkward position. Probably, he will not know the patient or the seriousness with which to treat these threats. It is unlikely in any case that he will be able to leave the hospital.

— Ask for the patient's name, address and telephone number.
— Advise the patient to call his GP.

— Failing that, advise the patient to go to the nearest accident and emergency department.
— If he refuses to do this, then inform the police.
— If the caller refuses to give any personal details, there is nothing you can do.

2. Assessment 1: What to do before you see the patient

AIMS
Collect information already available about the patient.
Make suitable arrangements to interview the patient.

COLLECTING INFORMATION

Most patients you will meet in a crisis or emergency are already known to psychiatric services, and this is particularly true of patients who present themselves to emergency services.

Sources of information

Sources of information include:

— Psychiatric case records to which all on-call medical staff should have access.

If these are not available, then other sources of information will become more important. These include:

— Key worker/therapist:
  • Psychiatrist
  • Social worker
  • Probation officer
  • Community psychiatric nurse
  • Hostel warden
— Medical case records.
— Ward staff who knew patient during admission.
— Ancillary staff:
  • Receptionists
  • Switchboard operators
— Voluntary agencies.

Remember that you must respect the confidentiality of privileged medical information (see Ch. 1).

PRACTICE POINT
The most valuable source of information is often the key worker.

You may learn that the patient has recently seen the key worker and a management plan has already been negotiated. It may be inappropriate for someone who does not know the patient to reassess him and alter that management plan. Most people would prefer a telephone call, even if it interrupts their meal, rather than be confronted with an inappropriate management plan (as they see it) the next morning. Even knowing who the key worker is may help you understand the presentation of the patient. Some people will attend in an emergency knowing of, or because of, the absence of their key worker.

Relevant information

The information you require is:

— Has the patient had previous psychiatric contact?
— What was the nature of the problem(s)?
— Is the patient in contact with psychiatric services?
— Is the patient in contact with other services?
— Has there been any recent change in contact?
— Is it commonplace for the patient to present as an emergency?
— If so, what are the usual problems?
  • Relapse of illness
  • Alcohol abuse
  • Break-up of relationship
  • Homelessness
  • Financial crisis
— Are there particular problems about such presentations?
  • Disturbed behaviour
  • Violence
  • Self-harm
  • Self-neglect
  • Poor compliance
  • Sexual disinhibition
— Were particular management strategies necessary?
  • Special nursing
  • Intensive care unit

- Medical problems
- Physical investigations
- Care of dependents

ARRANGEMENTS FOR INTERVIEW

Most patients presenting as an emergency are worried and/or distressed, regardless of the presence or absence of psychiatric illness (see Ch. 3: 'Reduce anxiety'). It can only make matters worse if the patient arrives to find he is unexpected, his notes cannot be found, or that no one knows when he will be seen. It is always important to plan for appropriate and safe initial assessment.

Inform other staff

In most hospitals referrals are made to the on-call doctor and other staff will have no knowledge of the referral. The first step is to assess which, if any, of the other available staff need to be informed of the arrival of the patient. During the daytime, reception staff will have to be informed to make a room available and may be free to find the notes. Out of hours, special arrangements will have to be made if nursing or other staff are required by the duty doctor.

Where to interview the patient

A suitably equipped interview room requires:

— Comfortable and sufficient seating.
— Privacy.
— Accessibility.
— Telephone extension or emergency bell.
— Desk and stationery.

It may be appropriate to interview a patient alone in an interview room knowing there are reception and nursing staff easily available, but it may not be appropriate to be alone with the same patient in an isolated room in the middle of the night. A useful additional resource is an open area with seats and a table which could be used if it is inappropriate to see a patient in an isolated room.

Seeing the patient alone

You must be safe and the patient must be safeguarded.
Moreover you will not carry out a satisfactory assessment if you
are frightened. Not only will this interfere with your decision
making, but it is quite likely you will communicate this fear to
the patient.

PRACTICE POINT
Always ask yourself whether it is appropriate to interview the patient
alone? (Spotting the potential for violence is covered in detail in
Ch. 9.)

It may be inappropriate to see the patient alone if:

— Presenting problem includes disturbed or violent behaviour.
— There is a past history of such behaviour.
— The patient is demanding a particular course of action.
— Your first sight of the patient suggests he may be violent (see
 Ch. 9).
— If the patient is accompanied by friends or relatives who
 exhibit these features.

It may be helpful to:

— See the patient with a relative or friend who can reassure
 him.
— See the patient with a professional or voluntary worker who
 knows him.
— See the patient accompanied by nursing staff.

Remember that relatives, friends or professional advisers may
be important informants and should not be allowed to disappear
from the hospital without your speaking to them, or having a
note of their names and a contact address or telephone
number.

MAJOR INCIDENTS

Serious violence or threatened violence is becoming increasingly
common in city hospitals which have open access (see Ch. 9). In
the most recent such episode in our own hospital, a patient left
the outpatient department and poured a can of petrol over
himself and the floor of a ward. He then threatened to light this
with a cigarette lighter.

PRACTICE POINT
Only attempt to deal with a major incident on your own if delay would result in life-threatening injury, e.g. patient about to jump out of a window.

When confronted by a major incident, your first reaction may be to rush in and help, particularly if a friend or colleague is involved. Usually it will be more appropriate to:

— Take a few minutes to plan a course of action.
— Inform the operator of the nature of the incident and where it has occurred.
— Discuss the emergency with a senior doctor on call if there is time.

Where violence to others or damage to hospital property is threatened it may be appropriate to call the police immediately.

PRACTICE POINT
All hospitals should have an agreed procedure for dealing with major incidents. This should include an emergency telephone number to alert the switchboard.

3. Assessment 2: Emergency history and examination

AIMS
Put the patient at his ease.
Obtain the necessary information about his mental and physical health to initiate management.

HOW TO START THE INTERVIEW

This is important. The patient's first impression of you often sticks. Try to remember that at the very least the patient will probably feel anxious, possibly even frightened or out of control.

Introduce yourself

Give your name clearly and address the patient by his name. Introduce anyone who is with you, e.g. medical student, nurse, and ask the patient's permission for them to stay. Direct the patient to a seat. If necessary orientate him in time and place (remember this may need to be repeated for some patients).

Reduce anxiety

Doing everything above will have helped. In addition the following are important:

— State the purpose of the interview and let the patient know that you will try your best to help.
— Tell him what you already know, e.g. a summary of what the referring agent has told you (be tactful in this regard).
— A statement letting the patient appreciate you have some understanding of his feelings may help, e.g. 'You must feel very worried about having to come here?'

Listening

Let the patient talk uninterrupted, at least for the first few minutes. Even if much of what is said seems irrelevant this is important. It demonstrates a willingness to listen and often yields useful information about mental state which guides the rest of the interview.

Reflecting

A reflective style of interviewing is useful. As the interview progresses tell the patient what you have perceived his main problems to be. This allows him to clarify key points and to confirm or refute your understanding of things. Again it also demonstrates that you have been listening.

WHAT TO ASK

Psychiatric emergencies can rarely be dealt with quickly. Proper and thorough assessments save time. Do not yield to pressure to act hastily whether it comes from patients, their relatives, or even colleagues. Keep the interview reasonably structured. That way important things are less likely to be omitted.

The history should aim to answer some key questions:

— What are the main current problems?
— What if any are the precipitants?
— Why is the patient presenting now? (as opposed to last night/week).
— Has the patient looked elsewhere for help?
— What help has already been given?
— What are the patient's expectations of this consultation?

In an emergency the history needs to be focused and the above questions should help you to do this. The following may also be informative:

— Past psychiatric history:
  • Is this presentation similar to previous presentations?
  • What treatment worked before?
  • Past history of self-harm
— Past medical history:
  • Does he have any medical problem which would explain this presentation?

- Is there any medical contraindication to your proposed treatment? e.g. history of heart block is a contraindication of treatment with tricyclic antidepressants
- Would drug side-effects or toxicity explain the presentation?
- Would the patient's drug therapy limit your treatment options because of possible drug interactions? (see Ch. 13)
— Family history:
- In an unexplained presentation does the family history provide clues about diagnosis?
— Personal history:
- What kind of problems has the patient had in the past? (See Ch. 4: 'Use of problem lists'.)
- How does he cope with these problems?
— Alcohol and drug abuse (see Chs 7 and 8).
— Social situation:
- Has a recent change in social situation contributed to the presentation? (see case history 3)

Clearly not all of the above information will be obtainable from every patient. Patients who have difficulty communicating or whose behaviour hinders communication will be discussed in Chapter 10. Information obtained from the patient should always be verified and supplemented by interviewing others, e.g. GP, relatives, if necessary by telephone.

PRACTICE POINT
Important informants should never be allowed to leave without seeing the doctor.

MENTAL STATE EXAMINATION

The following is a checklist:

— Appearance and behaviour:
- Evidence of neglect
- Is his dress appropriate?
- Is his manner appropriate?
- What is the amount of motor activity?
- Abnormal movements?
— Speech:
- Note rate, form and volume
- Does he answer questions appropriately?

— Mood:
  • Record patient's description of mood
  • Visible anxiety, depression, euphoria, elation or anger
  • Is it congruent with the topic under discussion and with facial expression?
  • How does the patient make you feel?

PRACTICE POINT
Never forget to ask about suicidal ideas (see Ch. 6).

— Thought:
  • Preoccupations
  • Delusions
  • Obsessions
  • Phobias
  • Circumstantiality
  • Answering off the point
  • Flight of ideas
  • Knight's move speech
— Abnormalities of perception:
  • Hallucinations (usually auditory or visual, but can occur in any of the sensory modalities)
  • Illusions (common in organic states)
  • Derealization and depersonalization

Cognitive functions

Testing of cognitive function in an emergency must be guided by the patient's age, physical condition and by the history, e.g. it would be more detailed in a 75-year-old presenting with memory loss than in a 20-year-old with phobic symptoms. During history taking in all patients:

— Assess level of consciousness.
— Be aware of any gaps in memory as evidenced by poor or inconsistent history.
— In all patients test:
  • Orientation in time and place
  • Short-term memory for a name and address after 5 minutes
  In the presence of any abnormalities fuller cognitive testing must be carried out:

— Test comprehension, e.g. ability to carry out simple instructions.

— Test logical memory, e.g. Babcock's sentence.
— If the above are impaired, test for localizing features, e.g.
   parietal lobe signs (see Departments of Psychiatry and Child
   Psychiatry: Institute of Psychiatry and the Maudsley Hospital
   London, 1987).

PHYSICAL EXAMINATION

Psychiatrists probably err on the side of doing too few physical
examinations. Just because a patient has been referred by
another doctor, this does not mean physical examination can be
omitted with impunity.

PRACTICE POINT
*Never omit a physical examination because the patient has been
assessed by another doctor.*

We have seen patients with subdural haematomas, transient
ischaemic attacks and even cardiac failure sent to our service
from other hospitals as psychiatric emergencies (see case history
11).

Remember:

— Physical and psychiatric problems commonly coexist.
— Physical illness may present with psychiatric symptoms (see
   Table 3.1).
— Physical illness may precipitate psychiatric illness.

Table 3.1 Physical illness presenting with psychiatric symptoms*

Illness	Psychiatric symptom
Epilepsy	Hallucinations, delusions, rage attacks, fugues, amnesias, mood changes, stupor
Cerebrovascular disease	Confusion, irritability, personality change, memory loss
Thyrotoxicosis	Anxiety, agitation, confusion
Hypothyroidism	Dementia, depression
Hypoglycaemia	Anxiety, confusion, violence
Cushing's syndrome	Depression
Tachyarrhythmias	Anxiety

*For a fuller discussion of the relationship between physical and psychiatric
disorder see Lishman (1987).

Table 3.1 is by no means exhaustive and gives only a few examples of physical disorders which may present to the psychiatrist. It should be enough to remind the psychiatrist that at the very least he should always ask himself 'Do I need to do a physical examination on this patient?'

The following groups of patients should always be examined:

— Patients with symptoms or signs of organic syndromes, e.g. disorientation, decreased or fluctuating conscious level, memory loss, illusions.

PRACTICE POINT
Never assume the drowsy patient smelling of alcohol is drowsy because of drink alone.
This amounts to negligence and can lead to disaster. Patients with alcohol problems get head injuries, subdural haematomas, hypoglycaemia and epileptic fits.

— Patients presenting for the first time in middle age with psychosis.
— Patients with possibly relevant physical illness — be guided by the history here, e.g. those with a history of diabetes mellitus, vascular disease or epilepsy.
— Anyone who requires admission should have a physical examination.
— Elderly patients — the association between physical and mental illness is greater with increasing age.

WHAT CAN NEVER BE OMITTED

— History:
  • List of current problems with precipitants
  • Past medical and psychiatric histories
  • Drugs — prescribed and non-prescribed
  • Alcohol
  • Name and telephone number of key contacts e.g. spouse, GP
— Mental state:
  • Orientation and conscious level
  • Memory
  • Psychotic symptoms

- ● Mood
- ● Suicidal ideas and intent
— Social:
  - ● Where will he go if not admitted?
  - ● Who will be with him?
— Should I perform a physical examination?

4. Management 1: Principles of emergency management

AIMS
Decide whether psychiatric treatment is needed and if not if there is anything else you can do to help.
Assess the need for admission.
Start an appropriate initial management plan.
Be familiar with the initial management of common psychiatric emergencies.

INITIAL QUESTIONS TO ASK

Does this person require psychiatric treatment?

If the person clearly has psychiatric illness the answer will probably be yes.

PRACTICE POINT
If after assessment the need for psychiatric treatment is unclear more information might clarify matters (see below).

Outpatient follow-up or hospital admission are options.

What kind of treatment is required?

Resist the temptation to rush into pharmacological treatment immediately.

PRACTICE POINT
The high level of arousal of some patients presenting as emergencies can lead to over-use of drug therapy.

Other options should always be considered. The following is a checklist:

— Reassurance and support.
— Brief psychotherapy (see below).

21

— Behavioural techniques, e.g. anxiety management (see below), breathing exercises.
— Crisis intervention (see Ch. 17).
— Treatment of relevant concurrent physical illness.

Where and by whom should treatment be carried out?

This depends on many factors. The kind of treatment being used is obviously relevant. Severity of illness is important, the mute depressed patient who is neither eating nor drinking needs to be in hospital, as do most suicidal patients. It is always useful to consider options other than admission. Most patients seen as emergencies do not require admission. (See below on 'Assessment of urgency of treatment and need for admission'.) Other options include the following:

— Outpatient follow-up (see Appendix 2: case history 1).
— Day hospital.
— GP.
— Community psychiatric services.
— Other agencies (see below).

For any given case other than those clearly requiring admission it is wise to go through this list before deciding how best to manage a patient. List the pros and cons of each setting for your patient and try to choose the most appropriate option.

If no treatment is required, how can I help this person?

If the person is not psychiatrically ill, but in need of help with a personal problem or a social crisis try to think of who else might be able to help. It may be appropriate to use one of a number of interested agencies (see below).

PRACTICE POINT
When you have decided on the initial action required it is important that this is discussed with the patient, his GP and the patient's relatives.

OTHER SOURCES OF INFORMATION

The answers to the above questions are often unclear in an emergency. Use of other sources of information is important in clarifying and completing the history. It gives you a clearer idea of the diagnosis (if illness is present) and certainly affords useful information relevant to type of treatment required and where it ought to be carried out. Sources of information include:

— Psychiatric and other professional sources (see Ch. 2).
— Friends or relatives who accompany the patient.
— Anyone who accompanies the patient.
— Professionals outside hospital, e.g. GP.

'Out of hours' there are times when it is wisest to contact the key worker or another professional (see Ch. 2). In carrying out this exercise the issue of confidentiality should be remembered. The patient's consent should be obtained if at all possible before he is discussed with anyone (see Ch. 1).

USE OF PROBLEM LISTS

The use of problem lists helps focus both your own and the patient's attention on which things are currently most relevant and which require immediate intervention. Along with the patient draw up a list of priorities and discuss how these should be tackled. Problems can be divided into psychiatric, social and medical (the three usually overlap). The following areas are important:

— Family:
  • Recent bereavements
  • Losses, e.g. children leaving home
  • Separation
  • Divorce
— Work:
  • Recent increase in workload
  • Job loss
  • Threatened job loss
  • Change of job
  • Change of colleagues
— Social:
  • Financial problems
  • Broken relationships
  • Moving house
— Medical:
  • Illness
  • Injury
  • Operations

PRACTICE POINT
It is helpful to find out how the patient has coped with previous problems.

Again the GP or relatives will have important information in this area. This allows you to assess a person's strengths and resources — reminding him of these is an important part of your management (see below).

USE OF OTHER AGENCIES

Ask yourself if you are the best person to be managing the problem at hand. It may be that the patient's family or GP could manage things perfectly well. Failing this there are many other agencies whose resources are appropriate for at least some patients presenting as psychiatric emergencies (see Appendix 2: case history 9). The following list is by no means exhaustive but gives some idea of what other agencies are available and when to use them:

— Councils on alcohol (see Ch. 7):
  • Useful when patient not requiring detoxification and for patients after detoxification
  • Individual or group counselling
  • Advice and literature
  • Social activities
— Social work departments:
  • Accommodation problems
  • Financial problems
  • Helplines (drug problems, rape, battered wives)
  • Day centres
— Self-help groups:
  • Premenstrual syndrome
  • Tranquillizer addiction
  • Single parents
  • Rape
  • Sexual assault
— Church organizations.
— Marriage guidance.
— Voluntary organizations:
  • Age Concern
  • Alzheimer's Disease Society

ASSESSMENT OF URGENCY OF TREATMENT AND NEED FOR ADMISSION

It is useful to have a checklist to consider when assessing urgency of treatment and the need for admission:

— How severely ill is the person?
— Degree of self-care (evidence of neglect, emaciation, etc.).
— Risk of self-harm? (see Ch. 6).
— Risk of violence? (see Ch. 9).

Admission is appropriate in the presence of severe illness, marked self-neglect or high risk of harm to self or others.

— What other support is available to him?
— Does he have insight into the situation? If not, and you delay admission or treatment, you may lose contact with the patient.
— How old is he? (The very old in particular may be less able to survive without immediate treatment.)
— Is he reliable with medication? If not, he may need to be admitted if there is no one to supervise this.
— Is the diagnosis or severity of illness in doubt? Admission may be necessary to permit the management of patients 'drug free' to clarify this.

The issue of compulsory detention often arises. The use of emergency orders under the various British Mental Health Acts is discussed in Appendix 1.

In summary, to be legally detained a person must:

— Be suffering from a mental disorder of a nature or degree which warrants his detention in hospital.
— Require to be so detained in the interests of his own health or safety or with a view to the protection of other persons.

'Threatening' to legally detain someone if he does not agree to voluntary admission is hardly within the spirit of the Mental Health Act and is ethically dubious. In practice if you doubt the durability of someone's consent and he fulfils the criteria for admission under the Act, it is preferable to detain him from the outset rather than threatening him with detention if he attempts to discharge himself.

EMERGENCY TREATMENTS

There is a tendency, particularly among inexperienced doctors, to rush to the drug cabinet in emergencies. This is particularly the case if patients are agitated, noisy or threatening. There are also many patients who demand drugs and this can be very intimidating for the doctor. The temptation to rush in with sedating drugs should be resisted. You should at least stop to ask yourself whether there is a genuine medical indication for their use. Many of the drugs used in psychiatry can be dangerous and sedating, and in certain patients (e.g. those with chest diseases and the elderly) can produce serious complications. The appropriate use of psychotropic drugs will be discussed at various points throughout this book. At this stage we would merely remind you that many patients, even when very emotionally aroused, can be managed by non-pharmacological means.

Non-pharmacological treatment

Brief psychotherapy is often very appropriate. This is particularly the case for patients with readily identifiable losses, or specific long-term difficulties. Brief psychotherapy operates on certain principles:

— It identifies the patient's strengths and prior level of functioning, and uses these to support the patient in the crisis.
— It is narrowly focused and problem orientated.
— The number and duration of the sessions is defined from the outset.
— It encourages appropriate discussion of problems and expression of emotion. Discussion of more peripheral issues should be avoided.
— The use of medication is discouraged (see above).

Simple behavioural interventions can be useful in emergencies, e.g. in management of anxiety or functional somatic symptoms. (See below and Ch. 13.)

FOLLOW-UP ARRANGEMENTS

At the end of any emergency consultation it is most important that clear follow-up arrangements are made. If there is to be no follow up, this should be stated clearly to the patient and to the referring agent.

PRACTICE POINT
Whatever your decision about an emergency referral, always record carefully your findings and the reason for your decision, for medicolegal purposes.

— The patient's GP should be informed as a matter of routine.
— It may also be helpful to inform others, e.g. social worker.
— Consent should be sought before doing this.

Occasionally you will wish to refer the patient to other specialist services which are better equipped to deal with the problem. What is available will vary from area to area. The following are usually available:

— Alcohol/drug-dependence services.
— Sexual problems clinics.
— Mental handicap services.
— Psychogeriatric services.
— Rehabilitation services.
— Other specialist medical services.

Details of how to refer to these services should be available to medical staff dealing with emergencies. If this is not the case in your hospital perhaps you could remedy this.

COMMUNICATION OF FINDINGS

It is both polite and necessary to explain clearly to the patient your findings and proposed plan of action. This is not always easy, e.g. with acutely psychotic patients, but some attempt at it should be made. Again it is important to contact the GP with your findings. Often telephone calls are helpful in addition to letters, particularly to GPs. This should be done promptly, although not always immediately (most GPs do not wish to be phoned at 3 a.m. to be told that Mrs Smith has been admitted). Remember issues of confidentiality when dealing with non-medical agencies. In communicating with GPs the following details are important:

— Diagnosis (if any — if not a formulation of the problem is useful).
— Suicide risk.

— Drugs prescribed.
— Action taken by you.
— Action you wish GP to take.
— Follow-up arrangements.

We have given examples of specimen letters to GPs in Appendix 3.

MANAGEMENT OF COMMON PROBLEMS

As indicated at the beginning of this chapter we have dealt with general aspects of management. There are, however, some very common emergency problems which are not adequately dealt with in other parts of the book. These problems comprise:

— The depressed patient.
— The psychotic patient.
— The anxious patient.

PRACTICE POINT
The two main priorities in the emergency management of these problems are:

— *To protect the patient from any adverse effects of his illness.*
— *To instigate effective treatment.*

It should be explained to patients that no psychiatric treatments work immediately and that most effective treatments take 1–2 weeks to begin to work.

Depressive illness

Admission to protect the patient will be necessary if:

— Suicide risk is high (the emergency admission of such patients is covered in Ch. 5 and the assessment of suicide risk in Ch. 6).
— There is evidence of neglect:
  • Unkempt appearance (see Appendix 2: case history 2)
  • Not eating or drinking
  • Marked weight loss
— There is lack of social support:
  • Homeless
  • No close relationship
In these circumstances if admission is refused it may be

appropriate to admit the patient compulsorily using Mental Health Act procedures (see Appendix 1).

Depressed patients with evidence of psychotic symptoms (delusions and hallucinations) should probably be admitted in the first instance. It is likely that they will require electroconvulsive therapy or combination drug treatment (tricyclics plus neuroleptics), both of which require close supervision.

Admission may also be reasonable if treatment in the community has failed. For example:

— The GP is no longer able to cope and he has tried a reasonable treatment for a reasonable length of time to which the patient has not responded.
— The family can no longer cope.
— The patient is deteriorating despite psychiatric outpatient treatment.
Other patients can be managed as outpatients.

Management

In all patients this will include:

— Explanation of the diagnosis and prognosis.
— Explanation of the treatment. This includes telling the patient that the treatment will not work immediately. It also includes warning patients about drug side-effects. The usual initial treatment will be a tricyclic antidepressant like amitriptyline or imipramine. Newer drugs, e.g. lofepramine, have fewer side-effects and for this reason may be better tolerated by some patients.
— Managing urgent social and psychological problems:
  • Helping dependent relatives
  • Dealing with housing problems
  • Dealing with problem relationships

This is very important and failure to take cognizance of these factors is one important reason for non-response to physical methods of treatment. Finally, if the patient is not admitted, adequate follow-up arrangements should be made including:

— Early outpatient appointment (see Appendix 2: case history 1).
— Communication with GP. He will remain responsible if the

patient is not admitted and will probably be the person who will institute antidepressant treatment.

Acute psychosis

Psychotic symptoms may appear in the following:

— Schizophrenia.
— Mania.
— Severe depression.
— Acute confusional states (see Ch. 13).
— Dementia (see Ch. 14).
— Drug-induced psychosis (see Ch. 8).
— Alcohol abuse (see Ch. 7).

The management of psychosis due to organic causes, drugs and alcohol is covered elsewhere.

Admission to protect the patient will be for the same reasons as in depressive illness (see above). In addition, admission to assess and treat the patient will be necessary if the illness is:

— First episode psychosis.
— A manic illness (see Appendix 2: case history 4).
— Associated with:
  • Socially embarrassing behaviour
  • Aggressive behaviour
  • Sexual disinhibition

If admission is refused by the patient the use of the appropriate section of mental health legislation to compulsorily detain the patient may well be indicated. Admission may also be reasonable if treatment in the community has failed for the reasons mentioned above in the section on depressive illness.

Management

Immediate management of an acutely psychotic patient involves:

— Explanation of diagnosis and prognosis.
— Explanation of treatment and its side-effects.
— Explanation of reasons for admission if this is being sought.

The details of drug treatment for the acutely psychotic patient are discussed in Chapter 5. In those psychotic patients not admitted intensive psychiatric follow-up will be required which may include:

— Outpatient follow-up.
— Attendance at a psychiatric day hospital.
— The use of community psychiatric nurses.

Finally, as in the previous section communication of the findings and management plan to the GP is crucial.

Anxiety

Anxiety is an extremely common presenting complaint. The first step in management is to decide the cause. Common causes include:

— Phobias with or without panic attacks.
— Panic attacks.
— Free-floating anxiety.
— Depressive illness (this often presents with symptoms of anxiety).
— Anxiety as a result of personal crisis (see Ch. 17).
— Anxiety as a result of disaster (see Ch. 11).
— Physical illness:
  • Tachyarrhythmia
  • Thyrotoxicosis

In the absence of depression or physical illness, admission is unlikely to be necessary.

Management

This comprises:

— Explanation of the symptoms, particularly if somatic symptoms of anxiety are present. Such patients often fear serious underlying disease or even death.
— Use of coping strategies:
  • Breathing exercises. Try to make patients aware of their breathing and help them control their respiratory rate. In patients who hyperventilate, rebreathing into a paper bag can be useful but can be dangerous in patients with cardiac disease or chest disease.
  • Relaxation techniques. The patient can be taught simple

relaxation techniques, e.g. he can be told to lie down in a quiet place, close his eyes, relax various muscle groups one after the other, slow down his breathing.
• Self-coping statements. In an emergency this may merely take the form of written statements from the doctor reminding the patient what he has told him about his symptoms and their management, and telling the patient to read these statements whenever the symptoms recur.

In general we advise against the use of drugs in controlling anxiety unless the patient's distress is overwhelming, in which case short-term prescription of a benzodiazepine can be used. Where physical symptoms of anxiety are particularly prominent the prescription of a beta-blocker if not otherwise contraindicated may improve some of these symptoms. The doctor should remember that he is unlikely to be able to fully abolish the patient's anxiety in one session. Follow-up is therefore important.

Treatment will depend on the cause of the anxiety. Spontaneous panic attacks will require treatment with antidepressants (both tricyclics and monoamine-oxidase inhibitors are effective). Phobias are best treated by behavioural methods. Free-floating anxiety may be treated using either behavioural or psychotherapeutic methods, and possibly also by drugs. Tricyclic antidepressants are helpful to some patients with free-floating anxiety and there is not the problem with dependence which benzodiazepines cause.

5. Management 2: The emergency admission

AIMS
Admission to the appropriate inpatient unit.
Liaison with nursing staff to plan immediate nursing management.
Plan immediate medical investigation and management.

APPROPRIATE INPATIENT UNIT

Once you decide to admit a patient (see Ch. 4), it will be your responsibility to decide which hospital or ward is appropriate using your knowledge of the local organization of psychiatric inpatient facilities. In the case of adult general psychiatry, most hospitals are organized in such a way that a ward team is responsible for a set geographical catchment area or sector. (The hospital should have a rota of wards who will admit patients of no fixed abode or from outside the hospital's catchment area.)

PRACTICE POINT
Always ask yourself whether the catchment area ward is the appropriate facility for the patient.

You should consider:

— Do the patient's medical problems necessitate admission to a medical ward:
  • Acute confusional state
  • Serious medical illness
  • Drug overdose
  • Serious self-injury
  • Urgent or sophisticated physical investigation
— Are there personal features about the patient that would make admission to a different psychiatric hospital desirable:

- Member of staff
- Relative of member of staff
— Or a different psychiatric ward:
  - Relative already in acute ward
  - Problematic relationship with fellow patient
  - Problematic relationship with ward staff, e.g. past history of assault upon a nurse
— Does the patient's age suggest he would be more appropriate in an adolescent or psychogeriatric unit?
— Does the patient have specific problems that would be better managed in a specialist unit?
  - Mother and baby
  - Alcohol
  - Drug abuse
— Can the patient be managed appropriately on the admission ward?
  - Violent or disturbed behaviour
  - High risk of self-harm
  - Sufficient nursing staff for his needs

LIAISON WITH NURSING STAFF

Ward nursing staff will expect to have an adequate amount of information about the patient:

— Means of referral.
— Reasons for admission.
— Problem list.
— Immediate treatment plan.
— Degree of nursing observation required.
— Degree of suicidal risk.
— Any special requirements, e.g. diet, assistance in walking.
— Infection risk, e.g. hepatitis B, human immunodeficiency virus (HIV).
— Legal status of the patient.

Suicide risk

The risk or threat of suicide causes much anxiety amongst ward staff. Admission to hospital is not a safeguard in itself. The most important preventative measure in such cases is to make a personal relationship with the patient. It is not surprising then that ward staff may be particularly worried about someone they have only just met and to whom they have had no chance to talk. Nursing staff will require the admitting doctor to be quite explicit about the level of nursing supervision required. The doctor should record this in the notes.

PRACTICE POINT
Written descriptions of the various levels of nursing observation must be available in all admitting wards. All staff should read these and agree about their meaning.

In most hospitals there is an official nursing hierarchy of supervision which rises from routine observation, through not being allowed to leave the ward unaccompanied, to special observation when the patient is never left alone. The appropriate level of nursing supervision will be a balance between the provision of a safe environment for the patient and the distress that may be caused by such intrusion. An additional contemporary problem may be a lack of trained nursing staff, or the presence on the ward of similar patients already.

Legal status of the patient

Most patients enter a psychiatric hospital as a voluntary or an informal patient. However, there are voluntary patients for whom compulsory detention would be appropriate if they refused to remain in hospital. (See Appendix 1 for use of compulsory powers.) Occasionally such patients agree to admission but because of indecision or having a dislike of the ward, wish to discharge themselves shortly after admission. We have known patients who have remained as 'voluntary' patients but were threatened that if they attempt to leave they will be put on a compulsory order. In effect this is using the compulsory powers of the Mental Health Acts but without the supervision the Acts demand.

PRACTICE POINT
Do not prevent patients leaving the ward by a threat of compulsory detention. The proper use of the appropriate Mental Health Act provides protection for both patient and staff.

Nurses of certain prescribed classes are empowered by mental health legislation to detain patients in hospital pending the arrival of a doctor (see Appendix 1).

INITIAL MANAGEMENT PLAN

The contribution of the admitting doctor to the initial
management plan will include:

— Liaison with nursing staff (see above).
— Physical examination.
— Instruction about physical observations by nursing staff:
  • Temperature/pulse/respiration
  • Blood pressure
  • Fluid balance
  • Food intake
  • Urinalysis
— Physical investigations.
— Drug therapy.

Physical examination

Some patients will have been physically examined as part of the
initial assessment. (See Ch. 3 for the indications.)

PRACTICE POINT
Any patient who requires admission should be physically examined.
Record and describe the presence of any bruising or other injuries
visible at the time of admission.

Disturbed patients

Some patients will be uncooperative on admission, and only a
limited examination will be feasible. The physical examination
will have to be repeated when the patient is more cooperative.

Victims of violence

In patients who are suspected to be victims of physical or sexual
abuse, do not carry out any examination which may prejudice
the proper forensic examination by a police surgeon (see
Ch. 11.)

Physical investigations

Remember that a patient who requires urgent and sophisticated
physical investigation is better placed in a medical ward. The

urgent physical investigations that may be indicated on admission to a general psychiatric ward include:

— Urea and electrolytes:
  • Dehydration
  • Alcohol withdrawal
— Blood glucose concentration:
  • Diabetes mellitus
  • Alcoholism
— Monitoring plasma drug concentrations in patients with possible drug side-effects or exacerbation in disorder:
  • Lithium — this must be placed into a plain blood tube with some estimate of time of last dose
  • Carbamazepine
  • Phenobarbitone
  • Phenytoin
— Blood concentrations of analgesics used in disguised deliberate self-harm:
  • Salicylate
  • Paracetamol

It may be good practice with certain emergency admissions to collect specimens for subsequent analysis during normal working hours, e.g:

— Urine sample for a drug screen (see Ch. 8).
— Blood sample for measurement of ethanol.

Drug therapy

PRACTICE POINT
Drug therapy should be kept to a minimum.

All doctors should be used to balancing the beneficial effects of drug therapy with the possible side-effects. The most important influences on this balance are the needs of the patient and these may change dramatically on admission. On the other hand the ward environment, staff and other patients need protection from disturbed behaviour. The removal from the stresses of the outside world and the provision of a supportive, caring environment are decidedly therapeutic.

PRACTICE POINT
Before you prescribe for a patient in an emergency, ask yourself if

this is because of a real need for urgent treatment rather than to calm the worries of those around the patient.

As general guidance we would suggest:

— In patients who present for the first time, do not prescribe unless there are clear indications, which should be recorded in the case notes.
— When a drug-induced psychosis is suspected, do not prescribe unless there are clear indications (see Ch. 8).
— For a well-known patient already in psychiatric care, it is reasonable to continue the drug therapy he received before admission if this has been well tolerated.
— In a patient with a well-documented past psychiatric history suffering a recurrence of illness, you may wish to prescribe on admission.
— A patient at risk of, or suffering significant alcohol withdrawal syndrome should be commenced on appropriate prophylaxis on admission (see Ch. 7).

DISTURBED BEHAVIOUR

Violent or threatening behaviour is not in itself psychiatric illness. (Violence and its management are discussed in Ch. 9.) Disturbed behaviour which is the result of psychiatric illness may be managed in wards with high staff numbers by non-pharmacological means. In most cases, however, drug therapy will be appropriate to alleviate the fears of the patient, and to protect both patient and staff. Although the emergency sections of the Mental Health Acts do not permit compulsory treatment of detained patients, doctors have a common law duty to preserve life and prevent serious injury to the patient or others.

PRACTICE POINT
Never force drug therapy upon an informal patient if there is sufficient time to invoke an emergency section of the appropriate Mental Health Act. Such management may later be construed as an assault.

As general guidelines we suggest:

— Always consider the oral route as the most desirable.

— Parenteral injection may be necessary if:
  • The patient will not comply
  • Rapid effect is necessary
— Always have sufficient medical and nursing staff present to prevent injury to the patient or any member of staff.
— If the disturbed behaviour is the result of a major psychosis such as schizophrenia, prescribe a neuroleptic:
  • Up to 200 mg chlorpromazine orally
  • Up to 150 mg chlorpromazine i.m.
  • 10 mg droperidol i.m. or i.v. may be less sedating. If ineffective, a further 10 mg can be given
— If the disturbed behaviour is the result of an affective psychosis, the above strategy may be necessary, particularly if the patient is not receiving any concomitant drug therapy.
— In patients with affective disorders receiving mood-stabilizing drugs, it may be sufficient to use:
  • Up to 10 mg diazepam orally or *slowly* i.v.
  • 2 mg lorazepam i.m.
— It may be appropriate to avoid neuroleptic drugs but use the above regimen of benzodiazepine drugs in:
  • Cases where the diagnosis is not clear
  • Drug-induced psychosis
  • The presence of medical illness when lorazepam is preferable because it is less likely to depress respiration.

Drug side-effects

All of the above regimens may produce excessive sedation, unsteady gait and hypotension. Neuroleptic drugs may produce pronounced extrapyramidal side-effects:

  • Sudden muscular stiffness (acute dystonic reaction)
  • Muscular rigidity
  • Tremor
  • Motor restlessness, particularly of the legs (akathisia).

See Appendix 4 for a fuller description and management.

PRACTICE POINT
Do not confuse drug side-effects with motor symptoms of psychosis. If side-effects are mistaken for signs of psychosis, then it is likely that the offending drug will be increased.

Serious drug reactions

Rarely a serious drug reaction is seen in patients receiving high-potency neuroleptic drugs which have usually been given in combination. This Neuroleptic Malignant Syndrome consists of marked muscular rigidity accompanied by fever and autonomic lability (marked fluctuations in pulse and blood pressure). It is probably more common in patients with concomitant physical illness and necessitates the cessation of all neuroleptic drug therapy (see Appendix 4).

6. Deliberate self-harm and suicide

AIMS
**Assess the suicidal intent of an act of deliberate self-harm.
Recognize which acts of self-harm are the result of
psychiatric illness.
Identify and protect those patients at risk of further self-harm.**

INTRODUCTION

The assessment of suicidal risk is one of the commonest clinical
problems in emergency psychiatry. Patients expressing ideas of
self-harm are seen in many different settings and referred from
many different agencies. For this reason we chose to include a
separate chapter on this topic. Since deliberate self-harm (or
parasuicide) is now one of the commonest medical emergencies,
we begin this chapter with the assessment of a patient who has
already harmed himself.

ASSESSMENT AFTER SELF-HARM

Interview

It is particularly important to find a proper setting for your
interview (see Ch. 2) and to remember the principles of how to
start an interview (see Ch. 3). If your patient is to talk openly,
he will need to be seen in privacy where you will not be
overheard. Such patients sometimes annoy medical and nursing
staff because they feel they are taking up their time needlessly
when it is better merited by the 'truly ill'. Even if a part of you
feels that way, you will not be able to assess the patient
satisfactorily if you cannot lay aside these feelings. Even if you
do not feel it, try to sound sympathetic.

PRACTICE POINT
If the patient is drowsy or confused, then a proper psychiatric
assessment cannot be carried out. Depending on the setting, the
assessment must be postponed or repeated soon.

Steps

The key questions of assessment in emergency psychiatry (see
Ch. 3) can be given a different emphasis. There are four steps
in assessment:

— Assess suicidal intent, i.e. was the act a serious attempt at
  suicide which failed?
— What was the reason for the act?
— Is the patient psychiatrically ill?
— Draw up a problem list.

Suicidal intent

There are three aspects to the seriousness of an act of deliberate
self-harm:

— The risk to which the person was exposed.
— Actual injury sustained.
— The likelihood that the patient meant to kill himself — and
  may still wish to kill himself (suicidal intent).

Suicidal intent does not always correlate with the actual bodily
harm inflicted. For example, a young man of impulsive and
violent temperament may react to a short-lived crisis by slashing
his forearm and causing considerable injury, yet an elderly
widower who takes 10 aspirin tablets thinking this will kill him
may be at much greater risk of a future suicide.

Measurement of intent
Suicidal intent is proportional to the number of these features
present (after Beck et al 1974):

— Preparation:
  ● Act planned in advance
  ● Suicide note written
  ● Action in anticipation of death, e.g. will

— Circumstances:
  • Patient alone
  • Timed such that intervention unlikely
  • Precautions taken against discovery
— Afterwards:
  • Did not seek help
  • Stated wish to die
  • Stated belief act would have killed him
  • Sorry act failed

What sort of patients kill themselves?

The assessment of suicidal intent is a guide to how seriously the patient wished to kill himselves. A complementary method to estimate the risk of suicide in the future is to be aware of the features prevalent amongst patients who successfully kill themselves. Completed suicide is associated with the following features:

— Demographic:
  • Middle or old age
  • Male
  • Divorced or single
— Psychiatric:
  • Previous act of self-harm
  • Depression or mania
  • Alcoholism
  • Antisocial personality
— Social:
  • Unemployed
  • Isolated
— Medical:
  • Any serious medical illness

PRACTICE POINT
The greater the number of these features present, the greater the risk of future suicide.

Reason for the act

Your understanding of what happened may be hampered by:

— Patient's embarrassment.

— Patient's unwillingness to disclose true motive.
— Lack of informants.
— The patient's mental state will have changed because of:
  • Passage of time
  • Effects of medical treatment
  • Alcohol/drug intoxication has worn off
  • A life crisis is passed or resolved — the self-harm may achieve this.

About one-third of people who deliberately harm themselves will say afterwards that they wished to die. About another third will say they did not care if they lived or died. When you learn of the patient's problems you may feel that other factors were important:

— Their feelings were hurt by another.
— They wished to express anger or hurt to important person.
— They were unable to cope with distressing feelings.
— The act provided an escape.
— The act brought them attention from others.

Such information will be helpful in drawing up the problem list (see below).

PRACTICE POINT
Always exclude abnormal beliefs which result from mental illness as a reason for self-harm (see below).

Is the patient psychiatrically ill?

PRACTICE POINT
Self-harm is not in itself a mental illness.
The majority of people who harm themselves have no psychiatric illness.

However, some acts of self-harm are associated with:

— Depressive illness:
  • Profound depression with suicidal ideas
  • Ideas of unworthiness or guilt
  • Delusions of wickedness or sinfulness
  • Hopelessness, i.e. negative expectations about the future

Hopelessness has repeatedly been demonstrated to be a major predictor of further self-harm and completed suicide — even more significant than depressed mood itself (see Beck et al 1985).

— Schizophrenia:
  • Ideas of persecution by others
  • Relief from hallucinations and/or delusions
— Alcoholism:
  • Associated with depression
  • Serious alcohol withdrawal syndrome (see Ch. 7)
  • Alcoholic hallucinosis

The possibility of the presence of psychiatric illness must always be considered when there is:

— A significant past psychiatric history.
— The presence of biological features of depressive illness.
— The presence of delusions and/or hallucinations.

Problem list

In view of the high prevalence of social and relationship difficulties amongst patients who harm themselves, it is good practice to draw up a problem list (see Ch. 4). Often this will contain important clues about the reasons behind the act, but, more importantly, it will dictate management (see below).

MANAGEMENT

Principles

The principles of management after self-harm are based on the general principles already discussed in Chapter 4. In the case of self-harm these will involve answering the following questions:

— Is the patient likely to kill himself?
— Does the patient need psychiatric treatment?
— What kind of treatment is required?
— Where and by whom should treatment be carried out?
— If no psychiatric treatment is required, how can I help this person?

Remember that for some patients the act of self-harm may be a solution to their problems rather than an indicator of continuing difficulties.

Safety of the patient

If the patient displayed a high degree of suicidal intent and/or has many of the characteristics of patients who go on to kill themselves, then the first step must be to keep the patient alive. Resources must be organized to support and protect the patient, and this may mean admission to a psychiatric hospital for assessment. (See Appendix 2: case history 5.)

PRACTICE POINT
Admission in itself is not a sufficient safeguard. The supervision and management of suicidal patients must be discussed and agreed with nursing staff (see Ch. 5).

In other cases this may mean the involvement of family and GP. Communication of your findings (see Ch. 4) to those involved may be an important management step.

Psychiatric treatment

Patients who are suffering a psychiatric illness should be managed in accordance with the guidelines given in Chapter 4.

PRACTICE POINT
The most important intervention in the management of the suicidal patient is the vigorous treatment of any psychiatric illness.

Compulsory admission to hospital

Occasionally you will meet patients who are suffering from a mental illness which requires treatment in a psychiatric hospital, and whom you believe to be at high risk of further self-harm or suicide, and yet they refuse admission to hospital. Reluctance to enter hospital may, of course, be a symptom of psychiatric illness if the patient is troubled by undue pessimism about the future or thoughts of unworthiness. In such circumstances compulsory admission to hospital may be required. The legal requirements for such an admission are detailed in Appendix 1.

Helping the patient to cope

For most patients the management will be about helping them cope better with the pressures of their life and assessing what steps, if any, might help reduce these pressures. This may involve the use of the skills of brief psychotherapy (see Ch. 4), crisis intervention (see Ch. 17) and involve some of the follow-up arrangements already discussed in Chapter 4.

PRACTICE POINT
There is little point arranging routine follow-up psychiatric appointments after self-harm. Only about one in three patients attend.

Severe mutilation
Rarely, the self-harm takes the form of severe mutilating injury, e.g. attempted castration with a sharp instrument, or the putting out of an eye.

PRACTICE POINT
Severe mutilating injury suggests the presence of a serious psychiatric illness and merits inpatient assessment.

Patients who repeatedly harm themselves

At least 20% of patients who have deliberately harmed themselves will do so again in the next year. A smaller proportion will do so several times. The assessment of such patients will follow the same guidelines as above. It should be expected that the degree of suicidal intent will vary amongst such patients and merits assessment. The reason for the behaviour may be:

— Response to a major life event.
— Response to a minor stress.
— Habit.
— Fathomless.

   As with most acts of deliberate self-harm, only the minority of such patients will suffer from a psychiatric illness. The management of such patients will again follow the guidelines above and will depend on the degree of suicidal intent, the presence of any features typical of patients who do go on to kill themselves, and the presence or otherwise of psychiatric illness. It is particularly important in such patients to adopt a problem-orientated management.

PRACTICE POINT
There is no good evidence that psychiatric treatment will prevent the repetition of such behaviour in the absence of psychiatric illness.

PATIENTS THREATENING SELF-HARM

Eventually we all meet patients who make dramatic threats that they are about to harm themselves or indeed kill themselves. You may be called to an accident and emergency department to see a patient standing in the middle of the room with a polythene bag over his head saying he is going to suffocate himself unless something happens. (See Appendix 2: case history 6.) Alternatively it may be that a patient threatens unless you admit him he will go out immediately and jump under a bus or the like.

PRACTICE POINT
No matter how theatrical these presentations may be, each must be assessed appropriately. It may be that such people do eventually kill themselves.

Assessment and management will follow the guidelines above. It may be helpful, however, to stress the following points:

— Remember what to do before you see the patient (see Ch. 2). Many such patients are already in psychiatric contact:
  • Has the patient got a key worker?
  • Has a management plan already been agreed?
  • Is it inappropriate to alter this existing management plan?
— Your assessment may be complicated by:
  • Patient's disturbed behaviour
  • The patient's demands
  • Your own fears
  • Anger and fears of other staff or relatives
— Try to set aside any strong feelings within yourself or in other staff and persevere with the assessment guidelines.
— In your management it may be helpful to:
  • Respond quickly
  • Appear calm (even if you do not feel it)
  • Sympathize with the strong feelings of the patient
  • Be directive in support of appropriate coping strategies and discourage inappropriate ones

After your assessment, it may be that you think it is appropriate to send such a patient home. You may even remind the patient that he is responsible for his own actions. You may feel you have done the right thing, but remain worried. Such assessment can be very stressful. Depending on your experience, it may often be helpful to telephone the senior registrar or consultant on call there and then, and, certainly, the management of such patients should be discussed at your regular supervision. This way emergency work becomes a learning experience (see Ch. 18).

7. Problem drinkers

AIMS
Be aware of the numerous ways in which alcohol-related harm may present.
Evaluate the psychological, medical and social consequences of drinking alcohol.
Exploit the patient's decision to seek help by a supportive attitude.
Recognize specific complications of alcohol abuse which require prompt medical treatment.

INTRODUCTION

The consumption of alcohol in this country has doubled since the end of the Second World War. The social and medical problems associated with alcohol abuse have risen in line with the increase in consumption. Problem drinkers can present at any time, in any setting and alcohol abuse may complicate psychiatric and medical illnesses. For these reasons we have devoted a separate chapter to problem drinking.

Terminology

In the past the definition of 'alcoholic' concentrated on the features of physical dependence on alcohol. Recent study has led to a broadening of the area of medical concern to include a wide range of alcohol-related problems. The two major components of the problems are alcohol dependence and the adverse consequences of drinking. *Problem drinkers* are people who are suffering significant social, medical or psychiatric problems as

51

the result of their drinking alcohol — irrespective of any physical dependence on alcohol. Common problems are:

— Psychological:
  • Depression
  • Anxiety
  • Suicide and suicidal thoughts
  • Insomnia
— Medical:
  • Accidents
  • Gastritis
  • Obesity
  • Impotence
  • Hypertension
  • Cirrhosis
  • Pancreatitis
  • Peripheral neuropathy
  • Cerebral atrophy
  • Epilepsy
  • Fetal alcohol syndrome
— Social:
  • Marital disharmony
  • Debt
  • Drunken driving
  • Absenteeism
  • Unemployment
  • Violence

In those patients addicted to alcohol, greater emphasis is now placed upon the behavioural elements of this addiction. The features of the *alcohol dependence syndrome* are:

— Awareness of a compulsion to drink.
— Obtaining alcohol becomes the most important behaviour.
— Increasing tolerance to effects of alcohol.
— Withdrawal features on cutting down (see below).
— Drinking to relieve withdrawal symptoms.
— Attempts to cut down drinking unsuccessful or short lived.

PRACTICE POINT
Be particularly concerned to question patients about their drinking when they have any of the problems noted above.

ASSESSMENT

The drinking history

The following information should be sought:

— Precipitants to referral:
  • Self-referral
  • Social crisis, e.g. homeless
  • Brought by someone else
  • Withdrawal symptoms
— Drinking:
  • How much in the last week
  • How much on the day of presentation
  • When and where
  • Consequences — psychological, medical, social (see above)
— Degree of dependence (see below).
— Other psychological, medical, social problems.
— Social or other support.
— Motivation for change.
— Previous experience of trying to abstain.

Precipitants to referral

Early intervention for problem drinkers is beneficial, but success depends on the problem drinker recognizing the nature of the problem and being concerned enough to do something about it. The precipitants to referral will often provide important clues about the problem drinker's desire for change.

Degree of dependence

It used to be believed that alcohol withdrawal symptoms only occurred after years in habitual heavy drinkers. In fact most problem drinkers experience symptoms of dependence, and typical symptoms are:

— Unable to keep to a limit.
— Increased tolerance.
— Early morning wakening.
— Meals missed because of drinking.
— Memory losses.
— Restless without a drink.

— Morning shakes.
— Night sweats.
— Morning nausea or retching.
— Morning drinking.
— Convulsions.
— Decreased tolerance.
— Delirium tremens (see below).

Motivation

Motivation is an ill-defined concept. It is not constant and it is very difficult to assess on one interview. Perhaps it is best envisaged as the patient's perception of the problem and his reasons for changing. Most experts in this field advise giving some practical test of motivation; e.g. arranging an appointment at a helping agency for the next day and asking the patient to turn up reasonably sober. (See Ritson 1986.)

MANAGEMENT

What to say there and then

It is important to support and encourage the problem drinker when first he decides to seek help. You may feel he has brought the problems on himself but it is important to be supportive and sympathetic. When hearing of his alcohol-related harm, it may be enough to say simply 'That must have been terrible for you'. It is important to reinforce the view that you agree he has a problem and should seek help.

PRACTICE POINT
In the absence of serious alcohol-related disability or severe dependence, most problem drinkers can be managed as outpatients.

The general factors which influence the decision to admit a patient to a psychiatric hospital have already been covered in Chapter 4. In the case of a problem drinker, admission may be indicated in the presence of:

— Past history of severe alcohol withdrawal:
  • Delirium tremens
  • Convulsions
— Severe alcohol dependence, e.g. drinking after-shave

— Concomitant psychiatric problem:
  • Depressive illness
  • Risk of self-harm (see Ch. 6)
— Lack of social support.

Set goals

Having encouraged the drinker to cut down his drinking, negotiate a change in his behaviour that can be accomplished by follow-up appointment. The goal might be to abstain until that appointment. Not only will this be a test of his motivation, but if he succeeds this will boost his self-esteem, and he is likely to experience positive feed-back from family, friends or workmates.

Involve spouse or family

The spouse or a family member will be an important informant and they are often willing to become involved in treatment and encourage the patient to change his behaviour. They are important sources of positive feedback when the patient successfully cuts down his drinking. Even a one-off interview with the spouse may allow the ventilation of angry feelings against the patient which might otherwise be turned against the patient in an undermining way.

Abstain or cut down?

There is debate amongst experts about which patients should be advised to abstain or simply moderate their drinking. If you have arranged an appointment with a patient, it is probably best to advise him to try to abstain until that appointment. The debate about whether they should seek controlled drinking or abstinence should be delayed until they are engaged in therapy.

Treatment of withdrawal syndromes

Patients likely to experience mild withdrawal symptoms are best advised to take time off work, to rest and to drink plenty of fruit juice or other soft drinks, but avoid large quantities of caffeine-containing beverages.

Patients who have experienced moderately severe withdrawal

symptoms in the past, may, in addition, be prescribed medication to minimize withdrawal symptoms. Benzodiazepines are the drugs of choice, and suitable initial regimens are:

— Diazepam 10 mg t.d.s.
— Lorazepam 2 mg t.d.s.
— The dose should be gradually reduced and stopped within 5–7 days.

PRACTICE POINT
Patients who have been dependent upon alcohol are at greater than average risk of dependence upon benzodiazepines.

In vulnerable individuals, benzodiazepines may, like alcohol, lead to disinhibition. Drug therapy for alcohol withdrawal symptoms is only essential in incipient delirium tremens, or where there is a past history of serious alcohol withdrawal symptoms such as delirium tremens or withdrawal fits. In such cases a higher dose of benzodiazepines may be commenced:

— Diazepam 10 mg q.d.s.
— Lorazepam 2 mg q.d.s.

Lorazepam is the drug of choice in severe alcoholic liver disease. If there is a strong history of withdrawal convulsions, prophylaxis with phenytoin may also be indicated:

— Phenytoin 150 mg b.d. or t.d.s.
— Continue for 1 week and then gradually withdraw.

Follow-up

Although the choice of agencies will vary from area to area, the choice is wide:

— Units for the treatment of alcohol-related problems.
— Specialist psychiatric services with a responsibility for treatment, training and research. Especially suited for patients with:
  • Severe dependence
  • Concomitant psychiatric problems
  • Those who have failed to change with other help
— General psychiatric units: these often provide treatment in the absence of specialist psychiatric units.
— Councils on alcoholism: these offer free counselling and

advice to problem drinkers and their families in a non-medical setting.

— Alcoholics Anonymous (AA): largest self-help group in the world where members meet regularly and assume that total abstinence is the only answer to alcoholism. The spiritual language may deter some patients from attending.

— Al-Anon is a parallel organization for the spouses and families of alcoholics. The family can attend without the problem drinker being a member of AA.

SERIOUS COMPLICATIONS REQUIRING PROMPT TREATMENT

Delirium tremens

This severe alcohol withdrawal syndrome only occurs some hours or days after the reduction or cessation of drinking and has a mortality of about 10%. The features are:

— Prodromal features of mild symptoms of alcohol withdrawal may appear earlier.
— Restlessness.
— Marked tremor of limbs.
— Disorientation in time.
— Often worse at night.
— Vivid visual hallucinations (often fearful).
— Suspicion, e.g. nurses trying to poison him.
— Insomnia.
— Autonomic overactivity, e.g. tachycardia, hypertension, sweating.

Management

Admission to hospital will almost always be necessary. Patients will be nursed as other patients with acute confusional states (see Ch. 13). In addition to monitoring fluid balance, electrolyte disturbance and blood glucose, high doses of benzodiazepines (up to 60 mg diazepam) may be necessary in the first 24 hours.

PRACTICE POINT
Concomitant physical illness is common in patients with delirium tremens and careful physical examination is essential.

Wernicke's encephalopathy

Wernicke's encephalopathy is believed to be due to thiamine deficiency and, if untreated, often leads to permanent intellectual impairment. Patients who die of this condition have haemorrhages in the brainstem and hypothalamus and degenerative changes in the mammillary bodies. The features are:

— Disorientation and confusion.
— Ocular palsies (particularly 4th cranial nerve).
— Defects in conjugate gaze.
— Nystagmus (especially horizontal).
— Staggering gait.
— Peripheral neuropathy.

Management

Immediate treatment by thiamine is necessary:

— Thiamine hydrochloride 250 mg i.m. or i.v.
— Parenteral administration of proprietary B vitamin and C vitamin injection (e.g. Pabrinex®, Parentrovite®).

If untreated, encephalopathy usually results in the residual Korsakoff syndrome when patients no longer have the ability to form new verbal memories and a progressive anterograde amnesia ensues.

PRACTICE POINT
There are many causes of acute confusional states (see Ch. 13) and these must also be considered when a problem drinker presents with disorientation or confusion.

Further information

Information on what treatment facilities are available nationally for problem drinkers are available from:

— Alcohol Concern, 305 Gray's Inn Road, London WC1X 8QF. Telephone number 01-833 3471.
— Alcoholics Anonymous, UK General Services Office, PO Box 514, 11 Redcliffe Gardens, London SW10. Telephone number 01-352 9779.

— Scottish Council on Alcohol, 147 Blythwood Street, Glasgow
  G2 4EN. Telephone number 041-333 9677 (for details of
  treatment agencies including local Councils on Alcoholism).
— The Northern Ireland Council on Alcoholism, 40 Elmwood
  Avenue, Belfast BT9 6AZ. Telephone number 0232 664434.
— The Irish National Council on Alcoholism, 19–20 Fleet
  Street, Dublin 2. Telephone number 0001 774091.

8. Drug-related problems

AIMS
**Enquire about illicit drug consumption during any assessment
— particularly in young patients.**
**Be aware of the management of drug-related problems
commonly presenting in an emergency to psychiatrists.**

INTRODUCTION

The taking of illicit drugs is not restricted to highly deviant
sections of the population, e.g. at least one in ten secondary
school children will have sniffed glue or experimented with
cannabis. Only a minority of drug-takers are addicts and it is
probable that most psychotropic drugs are similar to alcohol in
that they may be taken occasionally in moderation with no ill
effect. Most drug-takers will never see a psychiatrist and those
that psychiatrists see are more likely to suffer psychiatric, social
or medical problems. The taking of illicit drugs is usually a
phenomenon of youth. In contrast, the abuse of sleeping tablets
and analgesics legally prescribed by doctors is associated
especially with middle-aged women. The British National
Formulary clearly lays out the responsibilities of doctors in
minimizing drug misuse:

— Do not create dependence by prescribing drugs without
   sufficient reason.
— Do not increase the dose of a drug with dependence
   potential without good medical reason.
— Do not become an unwitting source of supply for drug
   misusers, e.g. prescribing addictive drugs to temporary
   residents.

61

ASSESSMENT

History

The information required in the assessment of a patient who abuses drugs follows the guidelines already laid down for the history of drinking alcohol (see Ch. 7). A few points, however, need special emphasis.

PRACTICE POINT
Most users of illicit drugs are catholic in their habits. Remember to enquire about alcohol, cigarettes, anxiolytics, analgesics, opiates, psychostimulants, solvents and hallucinogens.

Drug-related problems

The commonest problem found among drug-takers seen by psychiatrists is:

— Anxiety:
  • Acute, e.g. lack of drugs or fear of withdrawal symptoms
  • Chronic, e.g. because of lack of social skills or personality difficulties
  • Desperate anxiety may lead to demanding or aggressive behaviour

Other problems are:

— Psychological:
  • Apathy
  • Parasuicide
  • Depression
— Medical:
  • Withdrawal symptoms (see below)
  • Infection by hepatitis B
  • Infection by Human Immunodeficiency Virus (HIV)
  • Heavy consumption alcohol/cigarettes
— Social:
  • Crisis in relationship
  • Chaotic lifestyle
  • Convictions for possession of drugs
  • Convictions for fraud or theft (to obtain money for drugs)

- Unemployment
- Prostitution

Social support

Many people who take illicit drugs lead normal lives, but of those people seen by psychiatrists a disproportionately high number will have a history of social deprivation, disturbed relationships, and a lack of social support. This may well have implications for the follow-up of such patients, but, more importantly, it is probable that the major influence on people who take drugs is that of their peers.

SPECIFIC COMPLICATIONS OF DRUG MISUSE

Psychiatric syndromes that may result from the use or misuse of drugs are:

— Withdrawal or abstinence syndromes.
— Accidental overdosage.
— Intoxication.
— 'Bad trip'.
— Flashback experiences.

Withdrawal or abstinence syndromes

Drug addicts may present as emergencies in a distressed state and request supplies of drugs to combat withdrawal symptoms. Such syndromes are particularly associated with addiction to opiates, barbiturates and benzodiazepine drugs. In withdrawal from opiates:

— Symptoms increase in severity over 48 hours.
— Symptoms are unpleasant but leave no lasting physical ill-effects.
— There may be restlessness and sometimes fear.
— Physical symptoms are common:
  - Muscle and abdominal cramps
  - Nausea
  - Diarrhoea
  - Goose flesh
  - Sweating
  - Rhinorrhoea or excess lacrimation
  - Yawning

The abstinence syndrome in benzodiazepine dependence consists of:

— Anxiety.
— Restlessness.
— Insomnia.
— Variety of physical symptoms.
— Rarely withdrawal convulsions, especially in short-acting benzodiazepines.

The abstinence syndrome in barbiturate dependence is more serious and in addition to the features above may include:

— Vomiting.
— Confusion which may lead on to delirium.
— Withdrawal convulsions 1 or 2 days after dose reduction.

Management

PRACTICE POINT
In dealing with an emergency presentation, the psychiatrist must be cautious to ensure he is not an unwitting source of supply for drug addicts.

The psychiatrist should be wary of prescribing for strangers. Most drug addicts are successful in obtaining drugs without the help of a doctor. However, some drug addicts are skilled at presenting as an emergency with plausible stories which arouse sympathy. Management of the abstinence syndrome will be discussed again below.

Accidental overdose

A regular emergency in large city casualty departments is the unconscious young person who may be suffering from an overdose of illicit drugs or prescribed drugs taken in excess. The history may be obtained from an informant or simply inferred. It may not be clear until after resuscitation whether you are dealing with an accidental overdose or an act of parasuicide. Accidental overdose occurs when an addict changes supply, experiments, or has returned to drug abuse after a period of abstinence. Those who have access to illicit drugs may use these drugs in acts of parasuicide rather than drugs bought over the counter.

Management

The assessment and management of deliberate self-harm involving illicit drugs should follow the guidelines of Chapter 6.

Most people who have taken an accidental overdose will want to get out of hospital as quickly as possible. The counsel of perfection is that they may be more receptive to individual counselling at this time of crisis, e.g. how to reduce the risk of infection by HIV (see Appendix 5).

Intoxication

— Commonest psychiatric syndrome due to drug taking in the community.
— Commonest cause is alcohol.
— Most never seen by a psychiatrist or a doctor.
— Professional attention attracted by agitation, overactivity or aggression.
— Next most common is intoxication due to the inhalation of solvents:
  • Effects very similar to alcohol intoxication
  • Young males whose intoxication has led to aggressive risk taking
  • Found with a plastic bag or tin of adhesive
  • Glue on clothing
  • Perioral rash due to contact with solvent
  • Smell of solvent on breath
— In USA commonest cause of problematic drug intoxication is phenylcyclidine (angel dust):
  • Drunken intoxication
  • Concomitant confusion ('eyes-open coma')
  • Hallucinations
  • Can lead to murderous frenzy
  • Associated with homicide and/or suicide
— Intoxication by illicit drugs may be complicated by concomitant intoxication with alcohol and/or other drugs.

Management

Like intoxications due to alcohol, most gradually subside over a few hours. In solvent intoxication the initial effect may appear to be one of stimulation or euphoria but afterwards there is a mild hangover which may be accompanied by severe headache and nausea. There is no specific treatment. Deaths can be attributed to the direct toxic effects of solvents (e.g. cardiac dysrhythmias), trauma, inhalation of vomit or asphyxia (e.g. suffocation by polythene bag containing glue). Young adolescents will require supervision until the intoxication wears off. Aggression which is the result of drug intoxication may require some of the strategies discussed in Chapters 5 and 9. Chronic solvent abuse is not associated with psychiatric illness, but with social and family deprivation.

'Bad trip'

— Associated with hallucinogenic drugs which alter the experience of vision, sound and touch.
— Typically LSD-25 (lysergic acid diethylamide — 'acid') and, lately MDMA (methylenedioxy-methyl amphetamine — 'ecstacy').
— Leads unpredictably to marked emotional changes, e.g. terrifying sense of despair or anxiety associated with heightened perception.
— No deaths because of direct toxic effects.
— Risk of accidental death or suicide whilst perception is affected, e.g. jump from a height to escape some imaginary predator.

Management

A bad trip may last several hours and close supervision is required. 'Talking down' involves repetitive reassurance best done in a familiar environment by a trusted friend. The prescriptions of a once- or twice-only dose of a benzodiazepine drug may be appropriate, e.g. 10 mg diazepam orally. If disturbed behaviour is the result of fearful hallucinations it may be appropriate to prescribe a single dose of a phenothiazine drug, e.g. 100 mg chlorpromazine orally.

PRACTICE POINT
Once the bad trip has passed, the patient should be advised never to take hallucinogens while alone.

Flashbacks

— Spontaneous recurrence of part or all of a drug-induced experience.
— May occur up to 1 year after original drug taking.
— Most likely after prolonged use of LSD but may occur with other hallucinogens.
— Usually distressing.
— Psychotic experiences such as hallucinations may also recur.

Management

Protection of the patient and reassurance are the main aims. Usually symptoms pass in a few hours, but occasionally hallucinations persist and may require treatment by phenothiazine drugs.

DRUG-INDUCED PSYCHOSES

Chronic use of illicit drugs may lead to psychiatric illnesses which are indistinguishable from other serious mental illnesses such as schizophrenia. Drug-induced psychoses are particularly associated with:

— Amphetamines, cocaine, LSD.

Infection by HIV is also associated with acute psychoses, both organic and functional (see below).

The major features of drug-induced psychoses are:

— Marked paranoid beliefs, e.g. that people are out to harm them.
— Marked disturbances of mood.
— Visual, tactile and auditory hallucinations.
— Visual hallucinations may be prominent.
— Tactile hallucinations may be prominent in cocaine-induced psychosis.

PRACTICE POINT
The diagnosis of a drug-induced psychosis is not made on the clinical features alone, which may be indistinguishable from those of schizophrenia. The first step in the diagnosis is suspicion.

The presence of a drug-induced psychosis should be considered when there is:

— Recent onset psychosis in a young person (see Appendix 2: case history 7).
— History of recent alcohol or drug abuse.
— Past history of drug abuse, antisocial behaviour or prostitution.
— Physical stigmata of drug abuse:
  • Needle puncture marks in skin
  • Thrombosed veins in arms
  • Multiple sites of skin infection
  • Damage to nasal septum (cocaine abuse).

Management

PRACTICE POINT
The symptoms of a drug-induced psychosis are just as distressing to the patient as in an endogenous psychosis.

The management of such psychoses will be in accordance with the guidelines already given in Chapter 4. Most such patients will require admission to a psychiatric hospital. In the management of such cases:

— On admission a 25 ml sample of fresh urine should be obtained and refrigerated until subsequent analysis in a drug screen. Most major departments of clinical chemistry can provide routine assays for:
  • Opiates
  • Amphetamines
  • Tricyclic antidepressants
  • Phenothiazines
— In certain departments it may also be possible to assay:
  • Buprenorphine (Temgesic R)
  • Cannabis
  • LSD-25
  • Cocaine
— A blood sample for the subsequent assay of hepatitis B surface antigen and liver function tests may be indicated.
— The results of such tests should be communicated to the nursing staff.

PRACTICE POINT
The routine screening of drug-abusing patients for antibodies to HIV may be construed as an assault. Such an investigation should not be carried out without the express consent of the patient, and a thorough discussion of the implications of the result.

In the vast majority of drug-induced psychoses, symptoms settle within a week if the intake of drugs stops. However:

— In the interim the patient must be reassurred and protected.
— The staff, patients and environment of the ward also merit protection and disturbed behaviour may require drug treatment (see Ch. 5).
— As a last resort psychotic symptoms respond well to phenothiazine drugs.

PRACTICE POINT
Ward staff unfamiliar with drug-takers may have to be told that visitors may supply a patient with illicit drugs. Visits may have to be restricted, or supervised.

MANAGEMENT OF DRUG MISUSE

The management of the patient who uses illicit drugs has much in common with the principles in the management of problem drinking (see Ch. 7). Only certain points need be highlighted here.

What to say there and then

As with alcohol, most people who take drugs at some time in their lives will come to no harm. It is inappropriate to be alarmist with each individual patient where episodic drug-taking is an incidental finding on history-taking. Advice about the risks of infection by HIV are given in Appendix 5.

In those patients whose drug use is chronic and are seeking help, it is again important to be supportive and encouraging.

Information giving

If information-based counselling is to be effective, it must be done at a time when it is appropriate and the person is sensitive to it. In much the same way that good doctors remind their cigarette-smoking patients of the dangers of smoking, it may be important to remind drug-takers of:

— The dangers of the transmission of HIV by sharing needles:
  • If a patient is reluctant to cease intravenous injection, he should be advised where he can obtain a supply of sterile needles
— The effects of drug taking on reducing fertility.
— The adverse effects of drug taking on pregnant women.
— Availability of local agencies which help drug-takers.

Abstain, maintain, or harm reduction?

The management of chronic drug abuse is a controversial topic. Until recently in the UK there were two main schools of thought. First, drug taking was a form of deviant behaviour which should not be sanctioned or supported by the medical profession, i.e. the patient must abstain. The opposing view was that drug addiction was an illness that was the legitimate concern of the medical profession. Prescription of controlled drugs was one form of treatment. The Advisory Council on the Misuse of Drugs has argued that the spread of HIV is now a greater danger to individual and public health than drug misuse itself. 'Harm reduction' has the aim of minimizing the risk of HIV spread by providing safe and reliable sources of drugs until individuals 'mature out' of their drug-taking habits. The debate is unresolved and cannot be discussed in detail here. Local practice and philosophy will usually dictate whether there is a general policy to advise patients to abstain or whether maintenance will be offered. The decision to start maintenance treatment with addictive drugs will rarely be made in an emergency consultation.

Notification of drug addicts

PRACTICE POINT

A medical practitioner must notify in writing the Chief Medical Officer of any person he considers, or has reasonable grounds to suspect, is addicted to any of the following substances:

— *Cocaine.*
— *Dextromoramide.*

— *Diamorphine.*
— *Dipipanone.*
— *Hydrocodone.*
— *Hydromorphone.*
— *Levorphanol.*
— *Methadone.*
— *Morphine.*
— *Opium.*
— *Oxycodone.*
— *Pethidine.*
— *Phenazocine.*
— *Piritramide.*

Particulars to be notified to the Chief Medical Officer are:

— Name and address.
— Sex.
— Date of birth.
— National Health Service number.
— Date of first attendance.
— Name or names of drugs to which the patient is or is suspected of being addicted.
— Whether or not the medical practitioner making the notification is prescribing for the patient.

Notifications must be made to, and enquiries can be made

— Chief Medical Officer, Drugs Branch, Queen Anne's Gate, London, SW1H 9AT. Telephone number 01-273 2213.

In Northern Ireland, notification should be sent to:

— Chief Medical Officer, Department of Health and Social Services, Dundonald House, Belfast BT4 3SF. Telephone number 0232 63939 ext. 2867.

Treatment of withdrawal syndromes

The treatment of withdrawal syndromes is another controversial topic. On the one hand prescribed drugs may become a source of supply to patients who misuse drugs. On the other hand, a few patients may need medication to help with severe withdrawal symptoms. It is wise to avoid temazepam and buprenorphine as these are commonly injected.

Drug abusers who are physically dependent upon barbiturates may suffer withdrawal convulsions on reduction of intake and will require a carefully monitored in- or outpatient programme of gradual drug reduction. Patients physically addicted to benzodiazepines may require transfer to long-acting drugs such as diazepam and then gradual reduction in similar programmes.

Follow-up

The choice is wide:

— Units for the treatment of drug addiction.
— General adult psychiatric services.
— 'Needle exchanges' — in some cities in the UK there are clinics where drug addicts who inject can be supplied with clean sterile hypodermic needles.
— Local voluntary agencies (see below).
— Regional long-term residential facilities for the treatment of drug abuse — e.g. Phoenix House.

Further information

Information on what treatment facilities are available nationally for those with drug problems are available from:

— The Standing Conference on Drug Abuse (SCODA), 1/4 Hatton Place, Hatton Gardens, London, EC1N 8ND. Telephone number 01-430 2341/2.
— The Standing Conference on Drug Abuse, 266 Clyde Street, Glasgow G1. Telephone number 041-221 1175.
— Health Education Service, 16 College Street, Belfast 1. Telephone number 0232 241771.
— Health Education Bureau (Eire), 34 Upper Mount Street, Dublin 2. Telephone number 001-762393.

PSYCHIATRIC COMPLICATIONS OF HIV INFECTION

Many psychiatric illnesses are disproportionately common among patients infected by HIV. Several of these illnesses may lead to dramatic, emergency presentations:

— Acute confusional state because of brain disease:
  • Primary infection of brain by HIV

- Secondary infection by opportunistic pathogens
- Cerebral tumours, e.g. lymphoma and Kaposi's sarcoma
— Behaviour disturbance because of AIDS dementia complex. Associated with:
  - Marked cognitive impairment, e.g. slowing of thought processes, poor concentration, poor short-term memory
  - Motor features such as unsteadiness and poor coordination
  - Behavioural symptoms such as withdrawal and loss of interest
— Psychoses indistinguishable from schizophrenia.

PRACTICE POINT
A detailed assessment of cognitive function must always be carried out in a patient with HIV infection or at risk of such infection who presents with a sudden onset of disturbed behaviour or psychotic symptoms. Many of these presentations will be associated with brain disease which will require urgent medical treatment.

It is also established that AIDS sufferers are at greater risk of:

— Suicide.
— Depressive illness.
— Psychosocial crises:
  - Terminal illness
  - Death of friends or lovers
  - Problems associated with homosexuality and/or drug abuse

PRACTICE POINT
Always consider the possiblity of an HIV-related psychiatric illness among patients at risk of HIV infection: homosexuals, prostitutes, drug abusers, haemophiliacs, or their sexual partners.

9. Violence and its management

AIM
Recognise potential violence in time to take appropriate measures for the safety of all concerned.

INTRODUCTION

In recent years there has been an increase in physical violence in a variety of situations where once it was rare. There are regular reports of assaults on teachers in schools, on staff in the Department of Social Security benefit offices, on social workers by their clients, on GPs by patients, on ambulance personnel and, in particular, on the staff in casualty departments. Frequently in casualty departments alcohol plays an important part. Psychiatric services are not immune from this trend, but it is junior nurses rather than doctors who seem to bear the brunt of such threats and attacks.

SPOTTING THE POTENTIAL FOR VIOLENCE

It is the early recognition of people and situations that might lead to violence that is of paramount importance. It pays to recognize and defuse a potentially threatening situation rather than to have to deal with violence itself. There are certain conditions that are associated with violence:

— Alcohol:
  • Intoxication
  • Delirium tremens
— Drug abuse:
  • Demanding drugs
  • Intoxication

— Personality disorder:
  ● Explosive
  ● Antisocial
— Psychosis:
  ● Paranoid
  ● Mania
— Organic states:
  ● Acute confusional states
  ● Frontal lobe syndrome
  ● Brain damage
  ● Epilepsy
— Pain and frustration:
  ● Prolonged waits in accident and emergency departments

PREPARATION FOR INTERVIEW

Remember what to do before you see the patient. This includes collecting available information, e.g. case notes (see Ch. 2).

Think of safety first and consider these questions before interviewing any patient:

— Is there any history of aggression?
— Has he been drinking or using drugs?
— On first sight is he obviously agitated, unsettled, demanding, loud or suspicious?

If the answer to any of these questions is 'Yes' follow these simple rules:

— Do not interview the patient alone.
— Do not take him into an enclosed space, e.g. small office.
— Have additional staff nearby.
— Do not be confrontational.

NON-CONFRONTATIONAL APPROACH

It is important that any patient is kept informed about what is happening and who everyone is. This is particularly important where information processing is impaired through intoxication or psychiatric disorder. The information may have to be repeated many times.

— Approach any patient slowly from a direction that will not cause surprise or alarm, i.e. where possible walk towards the

patient from the front rather than approaching from behind or one side.
— Stop at least 2 metres away to address him, i.e. out of reach.
— Speak slowly, clearly and with confidence. You must speak loudly enough to be clearly audible, but do not shout.
— Introduce yourself in a way that is easily understood: 'I'm Dr Smith. I'm the duty doctor', 'I'm the duty psychiatrist' rather than 'I'm the duty SHO'.
— Check with the patient that you have the correct name, i.e. that you know who he is.

From now on you should do everything you can to make an accurate assessment of his problems, his mental state and his needs without startling, provoking or antagonizing him. Adapt as far as possible to the way he wants to be interviewed rather imposing your plan on to him.

— Invite him to sit down, preferably in a low chair so that you are given more warning if he is getting up. If he says he would rather stand, do not force the issue — allow him to do so.
— Try to put him at his ease. This can be done verbally and through your body language.

Empathy

Try to be empathic and reflect back to the patient how he appears to you. For example, with a very frightened and suspicious patient it might be helpful to start with 'A lot of people find hospitals rather frightening places at first', or 'Many people are rather anxious about seeing a psychiatrist — is that so for you?'

Non-verbal cues

Non-verbal cues to consider are:
— Posture:
  • Sit well back in your seat, but upright. This signals interest without being threatening
— Look at the patient:
  • As far as possible leave note taking until later. This

shows that you are interested in the patient's story and allows you to keep an eye on what the patient is up to.
— Do not make sudden moves.
— Decide what key information you require for your decision making. You may only have a short time in which to gather this information. A restless patient or one who is easily distracted may not tolerate prolonged questioning. You certainly need to do a full mental state examination but might not be able to test memory in the usual way (memorizing an address) but will have to adapt your technique to the circumstances.
— Do not be aggressive, demanding or confrontational. In your anxiety to make an accurate assessment you may become more demanding and hence threatening than you realize. If the patient wants to smoke and you would rather that he did not have a lighted cigarette as a weapon, do not say 'Don't smoke!', or 'Put that cigarette out!' Try to be pleasant about it: 'I'm afraid smoking is not allowed in this part of the hospital', or 'I'd rather you didn't smoke just at the moment'.
— You are unlikely to win any battle. It is better to 'swing with the punches', i.e. if the patient has decided to do something, you may as well make the most of it — within limits. If he wants to remain standing then let him. If he wants to interrupt the interview by visiting the toilet, then get a nurse to accompany him. Not to allow this will lead to arguments and lack of cooperation with your questioning.
— Do not insist on anything without the support of staff to ensure that you can carry it out. It is no good telling a manic patient that he must not leave the hospital unless you have the staff close by to detain him if necessary.
— Explain your findings to the patient in simple terms and spell out your recommendations. Again be empathic.

MANAGEMENT OF VIOLENCE

Priorities

When it occurs, and fortunately it is still rare, violence is distressing to all those involved. The priorities are:

— Safety of the patient — to prevent him harming himself or others.

— Safety of other patients and relatives.
— Safety of the staff.

The protection of property should have a low priority. Each hospital should have a policy for the management of such major incidents (see Ch. 2).

Adequate numbers

Except in extremis, a patient should not be tackled physically unless there are enough people around to ensure that the patient can be restrained without harm coming to him or the staff. Ideally a plan should be worked out so that the restraint is coordinated and safe.

— One person should take each limb (two may be necessary for the legs).
— As soon as possible, the patient should be laid on his back on the floor.
— One person should supervise, ensuring that an airway is maintained and breathing is not restricted.

Once this has been achieved the immediate pressure is off. There is time to think and discuss the next move while the patient is still immobilized.

Drug treatment of violence

Violent or threatening behaviour is not in itself psychiatric illness. The drug therapy of violent behaviour which is the result of psychiatric illness has already been covered in Chapter 5.

Intramuscular medication should be given while the patient is still restrained. It is dangerous for the patient and others if you attempt to inject a patient who is thrashing about. You never know just who might receive the injection! Do not reduce the restraint, or allow the extra members of staff to leave until enough time has elapsed to be sure that the situation is under control. In an emergency, this action may have been taken on a voluntary patient to protect him or others. Violent behaviour as the result of drunkenness or frustration at not receiving drugs, for example, should not be managed by drug therapy.

Further management

In a mentally ill patient, mental health legislation may now have to be used (see Appendix 1). The patient may also need to be transferred to a more secure ward.

The police should be called to deal with patients who have been violent, but are not mentally ill.

PRACTICE POINT
Record every episode of violent or aggressive behaviour in the psychiatric casenotes.

THREATS OF VIOLENCE

PRACTICE POINT
Threats must always be taken seriously. Do not rush to discount them as 'merely manipulative' or 'attention seeking'.

Frequently threats will be of self harm (see Ch. 6). Sometimes these threats will involve a risk to others, e.g. where a man in an outpatient department threatens to set light to a can of petrol. Any resulting explosion and fire could harm others in the building. Other staff should be alerted and patients evacuated from the vicinity. The nursing officer will be useful in such an eventuality. An unhurried, non-threatening approach is again most likely to succeed. This will give time for others to plan what to do next, e.g. call the fire brigade, police or reinforcements.

Weapons

Do not tackle anyone wielding a weapon. Retire and summon reinforcements.

A CHECKLIST OF SAFETY MEASURES

Here are a few things to consider wherever you may be called upon to interview or treat potentially violent patients:

— Know as much as possible about any new patient before the interview.
— If in doubt interview him with someone else present or nearby.
— Use a room with an alarm system and with clear visibility from outside.

— Ensure that there is no item in the room that could be used as a weapon (heavy ashtray, wooden bookend, etc).

— It should not be possible for anyone to prevent you from leaving the room — the door should open outwards and not be lockable from inside.

10. Difficult patients

AIMS
Use all available resources to obtain adequate information in order to evaluate and manage patients who are particularly difficult to assess.
Be aware of the different negative responses which some patients provoke in the doctor and deal with these appropriately.

INTRODUCTION

Patients may be seen as difficult for many reasons. Broadly speaking difficulties can arise in the following ways:

— A patient may have difficulty communicating with staff:
  • Stupor and mutism
  • Fugue states
  • Dementia
— A patient may be aggressive or violent (see Ch. 9).
— A patient may be a regular attender.
— A patient may have social problems, e.g. homelessness.
— A patient may arouse strongly hostile feelings in staff:
  • Personality disorder
  • Alcohol abuse
  • Patients who somatize
  • Drug abuse

These difficulties may be encountered in the context of a variety of psychiatric problems. Some of these problems are dealt with elsewhere, e.g. dementia (see Ch. 14), patients who somatize (see Ch. 13), alcohol abuse (see Ch. 7) and drug abuse (see Ch. 8). This chapter will attempt to deal with the remainder.

STUPOR AND MUTISM

In mutism there is complete absence of speech. Informants must therefore be sought to obtain a full history. Mutism is usually associated with stupor in which there is absence of any physical activity. The differential diagnosis of stupor is large and includes both psychiatric and neurological causes.

PRACTICE POINT
Physical examination should be carried out on all stuporose patients to help exclude organic causes.

The main conditions causing stupor are:

— Psychiatric:
  • Schizophrenia
  • Depression
  • Hysteria
  • Neuroleptic drugs
  • Dementia
— Neurological:
  • Epilepsy
  • Lesions of frontal or temporal lobes
  • Diencephalic lesions
  • Parkinson's disease
  • Encephalitis
— General medical:
  • Hepatic encephalopathy
  • Hypo- and hyperglycaemia
  • Uraemia
— Intoxication with alcohol or hallucinogenic drugs, e.g. LSD

It is often difficult to distinguish organic causes of stupor from psychogenic causes. The presence of purposive eye movements, response to commands and response to painful stimuli may be of some assistance but are rarely diagnostic. Table 10.1 provides guidelines on differentiating organic from psychogenic stupors.

In some stuporose patients muscle tone will be increased and there will be waxy flexibility and negativism. This is known as catatonia. It now seems to be rare in the western world. In any case, it too has both psychogenic and organic causes and its presence or absence is not particularly helpful diagnostically.

Table 10.1   Differentiation of organic and psychogenic causes of stupor

	Organic	Psychogenic
History	Clinical features suggestive of neurological or general medical disorder Psychiatric symptoms, if present, may fluctuate Sudden onset of symptoms Psychiatric features which are not typical of those usually seen in recognized psychiatric illness	Past history of psychiatric illness presenting in this way History of recent stress event
Examination	Neurological signs Conscious level may be reduced	Sad, hopeless expression Occasionally tearful
Course	Progressive	Fluctuates, sometimes improves
EEG	Grossly abnormal pattern depends on the cause	Probably normal wakening state

Management

Treatment depends on the cause. Admission will usually be necessary. Electroconvulsive therapy is useful in stupor caused by both depression and schizophrenia. It can however drastically worsen most of the organic causes and therefore should not be given until they have been excluded. If available electroencephalogram (EEG) and computerized axial tomography (CAT scan) may well add to the information gained from physical examination.

Stuporose patients may require feeding and rehydration and fluid balance should be monitored from the outset.

FUGUE STATES

These too have both organic and psychogenic causes.

Psychogenic fugue

Features of psychogenic fugue include:

— Narrowing of the field of consciousness, e.g. loss of personal identity (new identity may be assumed).

— Wandering away from normal surroundings.
— Subsequent amnesia for the event.
— May last hours to weeks.
— They are usually alert and aware of their surroundings.
— Behaviour usually goal directed and appropriate.

The commonest psychogenic causes are hysterical dissociative states and depression. Hysterical fugues nearly always follow some severe environmental stressor and often provide clear secondary gain, e.g. avoidance of marriage, avoidance of court appearance. As with other hysterical syndromes they should be diagnosed with caution.

Organic fugue

In organic fugues:

— Behaviour is more erratic and less purposeful.
— The patient may appear intoxicated.
— Organic fugues are usually of shorter duration.
— Conversation is likely to be more limited than in psychogenic fugue.

The chief diagnoses to be considered are epilepsy, head injury and intoxication. EEG is rarely feasible during the actual fugue state.

As with stupor, physical examination is imperative.

Informants need to be sought to get an independent history which may be helpful diagnostically, e.g. there may be a history of epilepsy.

Management

Emergency management of fugue states is difficult and patients should be admitted for observation and further assessment. Procedures such as sodium amytal abreaction although they may be useful, should not be done as an emergency. Organic brain disease needs to be excluded first and, in any case, abreaction yields best results in experienced hands.

REGULAR ATTENDERS

Every emergency service be it a general or a psychiatric hospital will be familiar with a number of patients who repeatedly present themselves. There are many categories of 'regulars' but the following are the commonest:

— Chronic schizophrenics — often attend looking for shelter, food, evaluation of physical symptoms or even just for a chat. They may be unable or unwilling to use other facilities.
— The homeless (see below).
— Abusers of drugs and alcohol — may attend for medications, treatment of withdrawal or demanding admission (see Ch. 7 and 8).
— Personality disorder (see below).
— Patients with unidentified psychiatric illness. It behoves us to remember this category.
— Munchausen's syndrome (see Ch. 13).

Some patients continue to attend because they are ill and illness has been missed. Those with previous diagnoses of 'personality disorder' may be dismissed after inadequate evaluation. Depression is particularly commonly overlooked. The authors also have experience of more than one patient with so-called 'hysterical personality disorder' who has gone on to have an episode of mania or a depressive illness.

Management

Principles of dealing with repeaters include:
— Discussion with the doctor who knows them best and careful reading of old notes. This is particularly important as some repeaters withhold important information, e.g. that they are seeing another doctor regularly, or that other services are involved with them.
— Re-evaluation of history and mental state. Chronic schizophrenics relapse, alcoholics get delirium tremens, patients with personality disorder get depressed. Do not dismiss people after a cursory glance at the old notes.
— Consider other resources which may be able to help, e.g. social work, voluntary organization, council on alcoholism (see Ch. 4).
— Set limits:
  • This must be done consistently.
  • It must involve discussion with other involved staff.
  • It will include discussion about the amount of staff contact which is permissible.

- It may stipulate conditions which the patient has to fulfil in order to be seen further.
— Look for any change in the style, frequency, symptom pattern and behaviour of repeaters. This may herald some change in his condition. Always ask yourself the question:
- 'Am I missing psychiatric illness here'?

HOMELESSNESS

This is not limited to any one kind of patient. Many homeless people present to emergency medical services because they don't know where else to go, or because they have had contact with that service due to previous illness. They rarely constitute emergencies but often have a wide range of social problems. Psychiatric patients are over-represented in this group including:

— Those with alcohol problems.
— Chronic schizophrenics.
— Those with 'personality disorders'.
— Increasingly commonly, the demented elderly.

Assessment

As with repeaters these patients must not be dismissed as 'social problems' after cursory and inadequate examination. A full assessment must be carried out. Important aspects of this are:

— History:
  - Why has the problem occurred now?
  - Has the person become ill?
  - Have previous supports been withdrawn?
— Mental state:
  - Is there evidence of depression?
  - Is there any cognitive impairment?
  - Is there a risk of suicide?
  - What is his insight/judgement like?
— Enquiry about what other resources (if any) have been explored.

Management

This will involve:

— Treating any illness, psychiatric or physical.

— Involving other agencies, e.g. social work, night shelters, old folks' homes, landlords known to be helpful. This can be notoriously difficult out of 'normal' working hours.

All emergency services should have a list of such facilities and how to contact them by day and by night. If your service has no such list, do something about it now.

PERSONALITY DISORDERS

Introduction

We have left this rather nebulous and difficult category until last. Any psychiatrist will be aware that there is much controversy surrounding the term 'personality disorder'; some psychiatrists even advocate that the term should be abandoned. Such arguments are beyond the scope of this book. Although diagnoses of personality disorder appear commonly in the notes of patients presenting as emergencies, we would advise against making this diagnosis on the basis of a 'one-off' assessment.

Definitions of personality are difficult but most include the idea of a set of attitudes, behavioural characteristics and emotional responses which are enduring to some degree and which are revealed in how we relate to others and to our social environment. It therefore should be obvious that 30 minutes spent with someone in an emergency department does not allow adequate assessment of personality to be made. Of course we may have case notes and other informants to help in the assessment but we ought to beware arriving at premature judgements on people seen once, and at a time of crisis.

All this being said, some people clearly do seem to have abnormal personalities as evidenced by difficulties in relationships, work and domestic life which seem quite consistent over time. Such people often present to emergency services after some crisis. Common modes of presentation include:

— Threats of suicide (see Ch. 6).
— Social crises (see above and Chs 4 and 17).
— Violent behaviour (see Ch. 9).
— Alcohol- and drug-related problems (see Chs 7 and 8).
— Factitious syndromes (see Ch. 13).

These patients often irritate staff (see next section) and this may in turn result in inappropriate management.

Assessment

In assessment rather than looking for features of particular personality types, e.g. histrionic, sociopathic, obsessional, a problem-orientated approach is better. Try to find out what precipitated the current request for help.

The following should be evaluated:

— Who is currently supporting this person:
  • Family and friends
  • Social work department
  • Doctors, e.g. GP, psychiatrist
  • Voluntary agencies
— What are each of these persons doing and could anyone do more?
— Is this person psychiatrically ill? Remember people with abnormal personalities also get psychiatric illnesses and indeed may be at increased risk of this.
— What does the patient want from this referral? He may want something you cannot provide, e.g. money or rehousing.

It is useful for doctor and patient together to draw up a list of problems which the patient should be asked to place in order of priority. This is a useful strategy before drawing up a management plan.

Management

This is usually multifaceted and involves:

— Treating any concurrent psychiatric illness. Beware over hasty prescriptions of drugs. Patients may 'demand' these. If you do prescribe give only 1 or 2 day's supply then review the need for drugs. If possible get a spouse/friend to supervise any medication.
— Looking at what other community supports could be provided. Go through a checklist:
  • Community psychiatric nurse
  • Social worker
  • Self-help groups
  • Regular contact with GP
  • Help with children, e.g. nurseries, share-the-care, fostering
— Use of crisis intervention techniques (see Ch. 17).

— Admission:
  - If warranted by psychiatric illness
  - If there is a real risk of suicide
  - If social support has crumbled and no other options are available

PROBLEMS FOR STAFF DEALING WITH DIFFICULT PATIENTS

We have pointed out that some of the above groups of patients provoke particularly hostile responses from staff. This is particularly true of regular attenders and those with abnormal personalities, who may make us feel angry and helpless.

Consciously recognizing and admitting this to oneself (or indeed to colleagues) is the first step to dealing with these problems. For junior staff in particular, talking to more experienced colleagues about such difficulties in supervision is important (see Ch. 18). We often tend to protect ourselves from our own unpleasant feelings:

— By projecting our own hostility and anxiety on to patients or their relatives.
— By rationalizing feelings by explaining them away or by intellectualization.

PRACTICE POINT
We should regard out own emotions as a useful clinical tool which tells us a lot about the doctor–patient interaction.

Taking all remarks made by patients personally is a particular trap. This goes for both negative and positive remarks. Beware of accepting flattery; it is just as likely to lead to errors in management as is over-reacting to criticism. For example, it may lead you to feel more responsible for a patient than you really are and therefore to become over-involved.

Awkward feelings about patients may give rise to other inappropriate management strategies. McGrath and Bowker (1987) list:

— Arguing with the patient.
— Condescension.
— Insulting him behind his back.
— Not listening.

— Premature discharge.
— Giving into his demands in order to get rid of him, e.g. giving him drugs.

To this might be added:

— Admitting the patient who annoys us. He often then becomes someone else's problem.
— Not arranging follow-up.
— Withholding treatment, e.g. to 'punish' people.

Appropriate responses to the difficult patient

The following are useful strategies in the management of difficult patients:

— Recognize your feelings. Discuss them later with colleagues (see Ch. 18).
— Listen and try to understand. Put yourself in the patient's shoes.
— Set limits. There are many articles on this topic including a particularly helpful one by Murphy and Guze (1963). See above: 'Regular attenders'.
— Avoid fruitless argument. Direct interview on to ways in which you can help, rather than going over irreconcilable differences, e.g. over admission.
— Use relatives or friends to help resolve difficult problems.
— Consider asking a colleague to see the patient. This should not be done to get yourself 'off the hook' but only if communication between yourself and the patient seems to have broken down irretrievably.

11. Victims of violence and disaster

AIMS
Be familiar with the range of experiences which can lead to post-traumatic stress disorder.
Be able to recognize this syndrome, make an initial assessment and begin appropriate management.
Be aware of the prevalence of various kinds of domestic violence and be vigilant in looking for it.

INTRODUCTION

In the last few months during the preparation of this book there have been two major air disasters and three major train crashes in the UK. Survivors of such disasters, and victims of assault and rape, may develop psychological symptoms which are distressing and disabling and which occasionally lead to more serious psychiatric disorder. For this reason we have included a chapter on the management of victims of violence and disaster.

POST-TRAUMATIC STRESS DISORDER

DSM-IIIR (American Psychiatric Association 1987) has a specific category called post-traumatic stress disorder. It has gained a prominent place in the American psychiatric literature but is relatively underrepresented in British textbooks and journals.

The core feature of the disorder is the development of characteristic symptoms following a psychologically distressing event which is described by the DSM-IIIR manual as 'outside the range of usual human experience'. Examples of such stressors would include:

— Natural disasters:
  • Earthquakes
  • Floods
— Accidental man-made disasters:
  • Fires
  • Road traffic accidents
  • Industrial accidents
  • Air crashes
— Deliberate man-made disasters:
  • Terrorist bombings
  • Torture
  • Military combat
— Rape.
— Severe assault.
— Threat to one's family.

Characteristic symptoms include:

— Re-experiencing of the traumatic event, this may include:
  • Recurrent, intrusive recollections of the event
  • Unpleasant dreams about the event
  • Suddenly feeling or acting as if it were reoccurring, reliving the event
  • Intense distress when exposed to reminders of the event or things which resemble it in any way
  • Guilt about surviving and about not having done more to help the others
— Avoidance of stimuli associated with the event or numbing of general responsiveness, as indicated by:
  • Efforts to avoid thoughts or feelings associated with it
  • Avoiding activities or situations which arouse recollections of the event
  • Amnesia for the event
  • Loss of interest in important activities, e.g. work, school
  • Derealization and depersonalization
  • Inability to feel normally for people
— Persistent symptoms of increased arousal:
  • Difficulty falling asleep
  • Anger and irritability
  • Poor concentration
  • Hypervigilance
  • Exaggerated startle response

- Physiological reactivity following events which symbolize or resemble the stress event

The DSM-IIIR manual states symptoms must be present for at least 1 month to be deemed pathological. Importantly it recognizes that onset of symptoms may be delayed for 6 months or longer after the event. It is also important to note that one does not actually have to be directly involved in an incident to develop the syndrome. For example, after a natural disaster such as a flood it is not only victims and survivors who are at risk but also staff on relief teams, emergency services and others who may witness the aftermath of the disaster. Those not badly physically injured are more at risk of developing post-traumatic stress disorder. Estimates of the prevalence of this disorder vary between 5% and 40% of the disaster population (all of these exposed to the disaster and connected with it in any way, see above).

It is almost the rule after any large-scale disaster that compensation claims will be made on behalf of the victims. For this reason documentation of their symptoms along with an account of their course and duration is exceedingly important. Some people may even need the label of 'post-traumatic stress disorder' to get compensation.

There is a body of psychiatric opinion which believes that psychiatrists ought to be more involved in disaster management. Such people believe that psychiatrists ought to be pro-active rather than re-active and offer wholesale counselling to all victims of disaster. This is not our view; we believe that unnecessary medicalization may create as many problems as it will solve. Psychiatrists certainly have a role in teaching other professionals to recognize the above syndrome. There is as yet little evidence that mass screening by psychiatrists to look for the disorder or prophylactic counselling of all victims is helpful. Not all victims respond by developing the above symptoms. Their response may be affected by:

— Underlying personality:
  - Strong or weak self-image
  - Optimistic or pessimistic
  - Wide range of coping strategies
— Presence or absence of psychiatric history.
— Social supports.
— Religious beliefs.

Post-traumatic stress disorder may be complicated by:

— Development of depressive illness.
— Brief psychotic episodes.
— Abuse of alcohol and drugs.
— Panic disorder with or without agoraphobia.

For this reason psychiatric screening of those identified as having the disorder is desirable.

Management

A wide range of treatments have been tried in post-traumatic stress disorder. These include:

— Drug treatments:
  • Benzodiazepines
  • Tricyclic antidepressants
  • Monoamine-oxidase inhibitors
  • Beta-blockers
  • Neuroleptics
  • Lithium
— Psychotherapy:
  • Individual and group therapy
  • Behavioural therapy
  • Cognitive therapy
— Hypnosis.

Most drug therapies only improve some of the symptoms, e.g. tricyclics and phenelzine relieve nightmares, flashbacks, panic attacks and anxiety symptoms. Beta-blockers relieve explosiveness, startle response, hyperalertness and other autonomic symptoms of anxiety.

It seems naive to think that such victims can be dealt with by merely physical treatments. Psychological therapies are essential. These include the use of:

— Grief counselling techniques (see Ch. 13).
— Crisis intervention techniques (see Ch. 17).
— Behavioural techniques:
  • Flooding
  • Desensitization
— Abreaction.
— Group therapy.

These may be used individually or in combination depending on which symptoms predominate in particular cases.

This is obviously a long-term exercise. Helping patients in the emergency situation involves:

— A listening ear.
— Use of drugs for prominent target symptoms (see above).
— Crisis intervention techniques.
— Arranging follow-up.

RAPE

This is common and grossly underreported. In addition to the sexual trauma and humiliation, the victim has frequently been violently assaulted. In a significant proportion of cases the assailant is known to the victim.

Rape victims may experience all the symptoms of post-traumatic stress disorder. Nightmares and reliving the event are particularly common. In addition, victims may feel intense feelings of guilt and shame. Rape victims may also isolate themselves from those who seek to help them, compounding their difficulties. Rape Crisis is an organization with particular experience and sensitivity in this area and victims can be directed to them. They will for example accompany victims who wish to report the assault to the police.

The following is a common sequence of events after rape:

— Numbness and shock.
— Phase of disorganization:
  • Anxiety symptoms
  • Depression
  • Inability to work
  • Inability to cope at home

This phase may last for months. Alcohol and drug abuse are a real risk, as is suicide.

— Phase of resolution and reintegration. This may take years.

Assessment

The initial approach is important as it may increase or decrease the likelihood of further acceptance of help.

It should involve:

— Considering who should see the victim. A female should always be present and if feasible a female doctor should carry out the physical examination.
— Acceptance as genuine. It is unusual for false claims of rape to present to emergency departments.
— A recognition of the victim's anxieties and some statements to this effect.
— The ability to tolerate anger, even verbal aggression from the victim, especially if the doctor is male.
— Explanation of why questions are being asked.
— Patience. Allow the victim time to answer.

Following this a physical examination should be carried out. This must be done very sensitively. If the incident is reported to the police, an experienced police surgeon may be available to do this. It goes without saying that careful records should be kept for medicolegal purposes, using the victim's own words where possible.

Management

This will need to be individually tailored. Principles include:

— Crisis intervention techniques (see Ch. 17). The ventilation of affect, especially guilt and anger, may be particularly important.
— Treating physical injuries.
— Contraception. Some women may request the morning after pill.
— Arranging adequate follow-up. Remember Rape Crisis again.

In any management strategy the victim's intense feelings of guilt and shame should be a prominent focus of the intervention. This is absolutely crucial in order to begin to restore self-esteem in the victim.

OTHER VICTIMS OF VIOLENCE

Victims of violent assault can be dealt with using many of the principles outlined in relation to rape. Doctors need to be particularly alert to the possibility of domestic violence including:

— Child abuse.

— Spouse abuse (usually battered wives).
— Elder abuse.

Problems of childhood are beyond the scope of this book. For an account of this important topic readers are referred to the recent Department of Health and Social Security publication (see recommended reading).

Spouse abuse

This is nearly always directed against women, although occasionally 'battered husbands' are found. Most incidents occur in the home and as with rape few are reported. Domestic violence often occurs in the context of:

— Alcohol abuse (in both partners).
— Poor marital relationships.
— Deprived upbringing. The perpetrators and/or victims may have been abused as children.
— History of other convictions (in the assailant).
— Jealousy.

Remarkably victims very often return to their spouses after the asault. In assessment of the victim look for:

— Substance abuse.
— Symptoms of anxiety or depression.
— Suicide risk.

Enquire tactfully about other family members, especially children. They too may have been assaulted.

Management in addition to the principles outlined in the previous section involves:

— Assessment of continuing risk. Wife and children may need help to leave.
— Use of social services/shelters for battered wives.
— Marital therapy (if feasible and the husband accepts the need for it).

Elder abuse

Sadly this appears to be increasingly common. It is often overlooked. Clinical features include:

— Unexplained or inadequately explained trauma:

- Bruises
- Burns
— Unusual injuries:
  - Bites
  - Injuries at easily concealed sites
— Injuries at various stages of healing.
— Evidence of neglect:
  - Bedsores
  - Filthy clothing
— Overconcern by relatives:
  - Refusing to leave the patient alone with you

Abuse may extend to repeated theft or fraud. The financial affairs of the elderly are often left in the hands of their relatives.

Having identified the problem the following are immediate priorities:

— Protect the victim from further injury. This may necessitate admission to hospital or local authority home.
— Identify any suicide risk.
— Treat any injuries.
— Arrange follow-up/referral to specialist services.

Finally, support to the caregiver is important. Abuse may arise when caregivers have been under severe stress from an increasingly dementing relative. This problem has been highlighted in several recent studies.

12. Psychiatric emergencies in casualty departments

AIMS
Interview the patient in an appropriate environment.
Take time to communicate effectively with casualty staff.
Assess patients appropriately in casualty, and take the correct initial steps in management.
Arrange appropriate follow-up if necessary.

INTRODUCTION

Although psychiatric emergencies constitute only a small proportion of patients seen in a casualty department (about 2.5%), they contribute disproportionately to the work of such departments in terms of time and by virtue of the disruptiveness of some of these patients. Such factors can reduce the efficiency of busy departments. For this reason we have included this chapter. We hope to point out that many of the problems caused by psychiatric patients in casualty departments are not inevitable and can be minimized by appropriate assessment and management, as well as by clear communication between all staff involved.

PROBLEMS FACING THE PSYCHIATRIST IN CASUALTY

Decisions made about psychiatric patients in casualty can alter patients' lives. For example, admitting a demented old lady to a medical ward because there seems to be no other option may result in her spending a long time there. It may in fact have been possible to manage her in the community or at a psychogeriatric day hospital. A telephone call to the on-call psychiatrist or psychogeriatrician will help clarify what is available and what is feasible. We elaborate on this point here to

101

illustrate that adequate assessment and gathering of information is essential to good clinical practice.

Site of interview

Most casualty departments are not built for psychiatric assessment. It is difficult to listen or to take a psychiatric history when the man in the next cubicle has just had a cardiac arrest and someone else is having a shouting match with the nurses. Likewise most casualty departments work under great constraints of time which may make the psychiatrist feel under pressure to make a quick decision. Hasty decisions lead to inappropriate admissions and discharges and should be avoided.

PRACTICE POINT
The psychiatrist must ask for a quiet, comfortable room to be made available. This is almost as essential to the psychiatrist for him to do his job properly as is a defibrillator to the cardiac arrest team.

Problems of communication

Unfortunately these occur all too frequently between psychiatrists and casualty staff. Often the reason is that neither understands how the other works. *Psychiatrists* should remember:

— Casualty departments are busy places, many patients require urgent life-saving decisions and action.
— Casualty officers do not have time to listen to a long psychiatric case presentation. A brief summary and clear communication of what action you plan to take is what is required.
— Casualty officers work shifts. The doctor who refers the patient may have gone by the time you get there. It is wise to get essential information at the initial telephone call (see Ch. 1).
— If the referral was inappropriate, check that the department has the information available to it to refer appropriately:
  • Do they have a psychiatric on-call rota?
  • Do they know policy on adolescent or psychogeriatric problems?
  • Do they know about emergency social work facilities? e.g. night shelters, hostels, social worker on call.

Casualty officers should remember:

— A proper psychiatric assessment takes time and requires appropriate facilities (see above).
— Psychiatrists do not have an endless supply of beds in which to place those with social problems.
— Not all psychotic patients need immediate admission (see below and Appendix 2: case history 3).
— Only a minority of psychiatric patients are dangerous.
— Psychiatric patients deserve as much respect and attention as other patients. The idea that some groups of patients, e.g. those who have taken drug overdoses, have 'brought it on themselves' displays a lack of understanding, leads to inadequate assessment, and to serious illness being missed.

Attention to these factors should improve relations between psychiatrists and casualty staff and hopefully lead to better assessment of patients. The psychiatrist should use the consultation as a (brief!) educational exercise. Casualty staff need reassurance about the behaviour of psychiatric patients, and clear guidance on immediate management.

The need for a prompt decision

It is rather ironic that much of the work in casualty departments is done by very junior doctors. It is also true that in many parts of the country psychiatric patients in casualty are seen by junior psychiatrists. When under pressure there is a temptation for all of us to make the easy decision rather than the best decision. There are many reasons for this:

— Medicolegal, e.g. fear of litigation if a patient threatening suicide were discharged and went on to kill himself.
— Criticism of peers. Patients seen in casualty are rarely reviewed by the doctor who sees them, be he casualty officer or psychiatrist. Fear of criticism may increase anxiety and lead to taking the safe decision, e.g. the decision to admit.
— Demands from patients and relatives.

These problems may lead casualty officers to over-refer to psychiatrists. In turn the junior psychiatrist will be more likely to admit those threatening self-harm, and may be less likely to admit other groups of patients because he feels he has to 'guard the door' and protect empty beds.

Possible solutions to these problems might include:

— Senior registrars or consultants could cover casualty departments.
— Senior staff could supervise juniors more actively (see Ch. 18).
— Juniors could be encouraged to discuss difficult cases with the senior doctor on call, e.g. patients threatening suicide and chronically psychotic patients.

MAKING DECISIONS

In this section we will offer guidelines only. Specific detail of how to treat different problems will be found in other chapters.

Major influences in decision-making in casualty (Gershon and Bassuk 1980)

— Current mental state and past psychiatric history.
— Dangerousness. To self and/or others (see Chs 6 and 9).
— What other supports are available? Can he use them?
— Is his self-care adequate?
  • Dress
  • Nutrition
  • Hydration
  • Hygiene
— How has he coped with such crises in the past?
— Is he motivated for treatment?
— What does he or his family want?
— Does he have concomitant medical needs?

Not all are relevant to all situations but they make a useful checklist for the psychiatrist in the casualty department. The following groups of patients have been found to be admitted more often:

— The old.
— Men.
— Single/divorced/widowed.
— Social class 5.
— Those perceived as 'dangerous'.
— Psychotic patients.
— Those with a past psychiatric history.
— Those with poor social support.

COMMON CLINICAL PROBLEMS

The following problems may present in casualty departments and be referred to psychiatrists:

— Alcohol problem (see Ch. 7).
— Acute confusional state (see Chs 13 and 14).
— Patients with unexplained physical symptoms (see Ch. 13).
— Self-harm (see Ch. 6 and Appendix 2: case history 5).
— Threats of suicide (see Chapter 6 and Appendix 2: case history 6).
— Psychosocial problems (see Chs 3, 4, 10 and 17).
— Antisocial or violent behaviour (see Ch. 9).
— Drug-related problems (see Ch. 8 and Appendix 2: case history 7).
— Anxiety states (see Ch. 4).
— Acute psychosis (see Ch. 4).
— Dementia (see Ch. 14).

It is worth bearing in mind that many of the above can present in a variety of ways in casualty departments. Some common examples are given below:

— Alcohol problems may present as:
  • Serious withdrawal problems, e.g. delirium tremens
  • Accident or trauma
  • Intoxication
  • Violence
  • Psychosis (a psychotic illness distinct from delirium tremens may be associated with habitual alcohol abuse)
— Drug-related problems may present as:
  • Violence
  • Withdrawal problems
  • Demands for drugs
  • Feigned illness, e.g. renal colic, in an attempt to obtain opiate drugs
  • Psychosis
— Acute psychosis may present as:
  • Disturbed behaviour
  • Bizarre physical symptoms
  • Hallucinations and delusions

13. Psychiatric emergencies in general hospital wards

AIMS
Be aware of and evaluate important psychological factors in patients with physical illness.
Be aware of the relationship between physical and psychiatric illness.

INTRODUCTION

Psychiatric problems in general hospital patients are surprisingly common. Surveys suggest that as many as 30% of general hospital inpatients have significant psychiatric morbidity although problems of classification and case definition have bedevilled most studies. In most general hospitals only 1–2% of patients are referred to psychiatrists. Most psychiatrists agree that this represents only a fraction of the psychiatric morbidity in these patients.

There are practical implications here. Not only are many psychiatric problems in general hospitals easily treated but they can affect the course of medical illness. Efforts to improve detection of psychiatric illness are thus important. Early detection may lead to better outcome for both the psychiatric and the medical condition, shorter stay in hospital, and reduction of emergency referrals to psychiatrists in a crisis.

PSYCHIATRIC SCREEN FOR PATIENTS ADMITTED TO GENERAL HOSPITALS

Psychiatric emergencies would arise less often if a few routine questions were asked of all patients on admission, allowing appropriate elective psychiatric referral.

— Recent life events (Creed 1985):
  • Bereavements
  • Job change or loss
  • Separation or divorce
  • Illness in family
  • Financial crisis
— Past psychiatric history. Include any admissions and treatment given.
— Mood:
  • Self report of mood
  • Appetite, sleep, sex drive
  • How does he feel about the future?
  • Does he feel hopeless?
  • Loss of interest in hobbies, friends, etc.
— Alcohol history (see Ch. 7):
  • How much? for how long?
  • How much in the last week?
  • When did he last have a drink?
  • Withdrawal symptoms
  • Offences related to alcohol, e.g. drunk driving
  • Time off work due to drink, e.g. hangovers
— What is his/her social support like?

PRINCIPLES OF ASSESSMENT

Many of the problems facing the psychiatrist in general hospital wards have been covered in the chapter on casualty departments (see Ch. 12). These include the need for:

— A quiet private interview room (if feasible).
— Adequate time.
— Proper communication with medical and nursing staff (often their views don't coincide).

It is often very useful to speak to the patients' relatives as well. After the consultation clear communication to all staff is important.

PRACTICE POINT
Even if planning a letter one should outline the important findings and management plan in the case notes.

COMMON EMERGENCIES IN GENERAL WARDS

Deliberate self-harm, alcohol and drug problems are covered
elsewhere (see Chs 6–8). In this chapter we cover:

— Acute confusional states (delirium).
— Patients with unexplained physical symptoms.
— Puerperal illnesses.
— AIDS-related problems.
— The uncooperative patient.
— Drug interactions.
— Problems of bereavement and the dying patient.

ACUTE CONFUSIONAL STATES

In general doctors are remarkably bad at recognizing acute
confusional states. They frequently misdiagnose such patients as
having dementia or even functional psychoses. This may lead to
inappropriate referral to psychiatrists accompanied by demands
to remove this noisy person from the ward. If these demands are
adhered to patients can inappropriately end up in psychiatric or
psychogeriatric care. About 10% of admissions to general
medical wards have acute confusional states and in those over 65
years old this rises to 30% (Lipowski 1983).

Acute confusional states are associated with increased
morbidity and mortality and lengthen stay in hospital. They
constitute a medical emergency rather than a psychiatric
emergency (see Appendix 2: case history 14).

Clinical features

— Altered conscious level:
  • Usually fluctuates
  • Attention and grasp poor
— Disorientation.
— Perceptual problems:
  • Hallucinations, usually visual
  • Illusions

PRACTICE POINT
*Visual hallucinations virtually always mean organic disorder (usually
acute confusional states, occasionally dementia).*

They are rare in functional psychoses.
— Agitation or restlessness.
— Sleep/wake cycle disturbed:
  • Usually worse at night
  • May be fine on the consultant's ward round next morning
— Short-term memory impairment.
— Affective changes:
  • Lability of mood
  • Fear and apprehension
— Behavioural disturbance:
  • Trying to leave the ward
  • Disconnecting drips
  • Aggression, usually verbal but occasionally physical
  • Inappropriate interference with other patients

Causes of acute confusional states

— Psychotropic drugs:
  • Benzodiazepines (ingestion or withdrawal)
  • Major tranquillizers
  • Tricyclic antidepressants
  • Barbiturates (ingestion or withdrawal)
  (N.B. Many of these drugs are used by doctors to treat acute confussional states.)
— Cardiac drugs:
  • Digoxin
  • Beta-blockers
  • Diuretics
— Anti-Parkinsonian:
  • L-Dopa
  • Bromocryptine
  • Anticholinergic drugs
— Other drugs:
  • Cimetidine
  • Corticosteroids
  • Alcohol (excess or withdrawal)

PRACTICE POINT
Very many drugs can cause acute confusional states. The above list is not exhaustive but includes some of the commonest drugs implicated. Always check which drugs a patient is on and consider any drug as a possible cause.

— Infection:
  • Any infection may be relevant
  • Remember HIV (see Ch. 8)
— Metabolic causes:
  • Electrolyte disturbances
  • All the failures, e.g. cardiac, respiratory, renal,
    hepatic
— Diabetic complications.
— Endocrine disorders.
— Head injury.
— Raised intracranial pressure.
— Vascular causes:
  • Transient cerebral ischaemic attacks
  • Subdural haematoma
  • Extradural haematoma
— Epilepsy.

Management

The following principles are important:
   Treat the underlying cause. This will always entail physical
examination and usually some preliminary investigations. The
precise investigations to be carried out depend on examination
findings but full blood count, urinalysis, urea and electrolytes,
glucose and blood gases make a useful initial screen.
   Appropriate nursing and general care:
— Use as few different people as possible to nurse the patient
  (this reduces the chances of misidentifications).
— Keep surroundings well lit.
— Remove potentially dangerous objects.
— Explain everything you do carefully to the patient. This
  may prevent a punch on the nose for taking blood without
  warning.
— Never forget to introduce yourself even if you have met
  the patient before (remember he may well have forgotten
  this).
— Repeatedly orientate the patient in time and place.
— Reassurance.

   As indicated above it is crucial to realize that much
behavioural disturbance is secondary to many of the more
frightening clinical features of an acute confusional state.

Drug treatment

The last thing you should think of is giving drugs.
Unfortunately this is the first thing of which many doctors
think. It is important to resist pressure from nurses in this
regard. Sedatives may lower sensory input and aggravate the
problem. They may also make matters worse medically, e.g.
giving diazepam to a patient with hypoxia, lowering blood
pressure with chlorpromazine.

In practice drugs are often required but think of all the other
management considerations first. It is inappropriate for a doctor
to sedate a patient for aggressive behaviour when that behaviour
has been precipitated by the doctor or nurse forgetting these
other principles. When drugs are required we suggest:

— Chlormethiazole 250–500 mg 4- to 6-hourly. If this fails:
— Haloperidol 1–5 mg 4- to 6-hourly. Some old people may
  need even less than 1 mg.

In a patient seriously at risk of harming himself or others:

— Droperidol 5–10 mg i.v./i.m. acts very quickly. It has a short
  half-life and may need to be repeated in 1–2 hours.

As a general rule these drugs should be given for as short a
time as possible. Chlormethiazole causes dependence and both
haloperidol and droperidol have significant side effects (see
Appendix 4).

PATIENTS WITH UNEXPLAINED PHYSICAL SYMPTOMS

Many patients in general wards have physical symptoms or signs
without objective evidence of disease. These patients are rarely
referred to psychiatrists initially but occasionally some crisis
precipitates referral. Examples are:

— The patient threatens discharge.
— The patient refuses treatment.
— The patient is causing a disturbance in the ward.

The psychiatrist faced with such a person in emergency has
three main tasks:

— To distinguish physical from psychiatric illness.
— To look for and exclude underlying psychiatric illness.
— To establish a therapeutic contact with the patient.

Distinguishing physical from psychiatric illness

Psychiatric illness should be diagnosed on the basis of positive features and not by exclusion. It is also important to remember that physical and psychiatric illness can coexist. The following factors may help distinguish psychiatric from physical illness:

— Symptoms are ill defined:
  • Vaguely described
  • Don't conform to anatomical or physiological patterns
— Symptoms may be prepicipated by stress events.
— Symptom severity is inconsistent with level of day-to-day functioning.
— The patient is often suggestible.
— Past psychiatric history may suggest underlying diagnosis.

Doctors often use the concept of secondary gain (the mechanisms by which patients obtain physical and emotional support from others from their symptoms) as evidence of functional rather than physical illness. This is a naive and mistaken belief. Virtually any illness, physical or psychiatric, results in secondary gain.

Excluding underlying psychiatric illness

Many psychiatric illnesses may present with physical symptoms. These include:

— Anxiety disorders:
  • Autonomic symptoms, e.g. tachycardia, tremor, sweating, dry mouth
  • Symptoms of hyperventilation
— Depression:
  • Vague non-specific physical complaints with hypochondriacal preoccupation
  • Chronic pain
— Schizophrenia:
  • May present with bizarre physical symptoms
  • Monosymptomatic hypochondriacal psychosis (single fixed belief of delusional intensity about some aspects of physical appearance, e.g. size of nose)
— Somatoform and factitious disorders. Classification of patients with unexplained physical symptoms who do not have an anxiety disorder, depression or schizophrenia is more

controversial. DSM-IIIR includes sections on somatoform
disorders and factitious disorders to cover these patients.

Somatoform disorders

These comprise:

— Somatization disorder.
— Hypochondriasis.
— Psychogenic pain disorder.
— Conversion disorder.
— Body dysmorphic disorder.

Factitious disorders

DSM-IIIR has divided up factitious disorders with physical
symptoms and factitious disorders with psychological symptoms.
The best example of a factitious disorder is Munchausen's
syndrome.

The key features of this syndrome are:

— Plausible and elaborate stories used to explain factitious illness.
— Wandering from hospital to hospital around the country
  seeking admission.

Patients often present with textbook histories, e.g. of
myocardial infarction or renal colic. They may go to great
lengths to fake symptoms, i.e. sticking needles in their urethra
to produce haematuria. A few are drug addicts seeking opiate
medications but most cases are not so readily explained.

Establishing a therapeutic contact with the patient

Often the most important role of the psychiatrist is to establish
enough rapport to keep the patient in treatment. Keep in mind
the patient may well be angry about the referral and see it as a
sign that he has not been taken seriously. The following are
important steps:

— Explain why you are being asked to see the patient.
— Listen:
  • Allow time for ventilation about the symptoms, previous
    investigations, management and previous doctors
  • Avoid colluding with criticism of other doctors

— Explanation and reassurance:
  • Explain previous investigations, diagnostic labels and
    treatments
  • Emphasize that you take his complaints seriously and
    believe his symptoms are real
  • Keep an open mind on the existence of underlying
    organic disorders but do not collude with the patient's
    belief in this regard if there is overwhelming evidence to
    the contrary
  • Reassure the patient that the referral does not mean he is
    'going mad'
  • Attempt to offer a reasonable psychological explanation of
    the symptoms. The use of words like 'stress' and 'tension'
    are helpful in indicating to the patient the relationship
    between mind and body.
— Tell the patient how you may be able to help:
  • Discuss areas of stress, e.g. work or family problems
  • Discuss problem relationships
  • The use of behavioural techniques, e.g. relaxation
— Talk about management rather than cure:
  • Don't promise total symptom relief
  • Aim at improving function, e.g. returning to work, going
    out with friends, playing sport again

For more detailed description of the above syndromes and
their long-term management the interested reader is referred to
the books by Ford (1983) and Kellner (1987).

PUERPERAL ILLNESS

This can be divided into three main groups:

— Baby blues.
— Puerperal depression.
— Puerperal psychosis.

Baby blues

This occurs in up to 50% of women. Usually peaks between the
third and fifth day postpartum. It may present as:

— Lability of mood.
— Episodes of tearfulness.
— Irritability.

It is more frequent in primigravidae and patients may have complained of depressive symptoms during the last trimester of pregnancy.

It is short lived and requires no specific treatment other than explanation, understanding and reassurance.

Puerperal depression

This occurs in 10–15% of women postpartum and is often overlooked. It usually begins in the first few weeks postpartum. Because it is missed so often, enquiry about symptoms of depression should be routine as part of postnatal examination. GPs and health visitors need to be alert to it as patients have often left hospital when it starts. Sometime other symptoms are more prominent than typical depressive mood changes. These include:

— Tiredness.
— Irritability.
— Anxiety.
— Overconcern about the baby (including unreasonable fears of physical and mental handicap).
— Fear of harming the baby.

The following are thought to be important aetiological factors:

— Past psychiatric history.
— Recent stressful life event.
— Younger age of the mother.
— Experience of postpartum blues.
— Poor marital relationship.
— Absence of social support.

Although most recover after a few months a significant number go on to have prolonged depressive illnesses making prompt diagnosis and effective treatment imperative. Treatment often involves a prescription of antidepressant drugs but psychological and social measures should not be forgotten. There is no contraindication to breast feeding while on tricyclic antidepressants.

Puerperal psychosis

The incidence is about one case per 500 births. The clinical picture may be that of an organic brain syndrome, affective disorder or schizophrenic disorder. It seems that about four-fifths of cases are affective in nature with an unusually high proportion of manic disorders. In addition to the normal features of the above conditions, the following are especially noted:

— Organic features:
  • Disorientation
  • Perplexity (this may be present even if the illness is schizophrenic or affective in nature)
— Delusional beliefs that the child is malformed.
— Threats or even attempts to kill the child.

Management

Early diagnosis and prompt treatment is important as both mother and baby are at risk. Treatment depends on the form of the psychosis. Admission is generally advisable, if possible in a special mother and baby unit or at least a ward which has facilities to cater for both mothers and babies. As with other psychotic illnesses it may be best to observe the patient for a drug-free spell to clarify the nature of the psychosis. In the longer term treatment may involve antidepressants, phenothiazines, lithium or ECT depending on the clinical features. If lithium is used breastfeeding is contraindicated.

The short-term prognosis is good but the relapse rate in subsequent pregnancies is 15–20%.

AIDS-RELATED PROBLEMS

This is mentioned briefly here to remind both psychiatrists and physicians of what will become an increasingly important problem. AIDS is associated with a vast spectrum of psychiatric disorder. This is discussed in detail in Chapter 8.

THE UNCOOPERATIVE PATIENT

Medical and nursing staff usually have views on how patients who are ill ought to behave. These views usually include the idea that patients should comply with treatment, acquiesce with decisions made in their 'best interests' and so on. When patients deviate from these norms some staff become anxious or even hostile.

A patient's lack of cooperation may stem from many causes:

— Fear. Usually related to lack of understanding of diagnosis, management and prognosis. This needs to be given in jargon-free language and on more than one occasion. Written information can be very helpful.
— Problems of culture and language.
— Mental illness:
  • Depression
  • Mental handicap
  • Psychosis

These all impair judgement and understanding.

Management

This will depend on which of the above causes prevails. Some of the guidelines given in the section on managing patients with unexplained physical symptoms are relevant (see also Ch. 10).

DRUG INTERACTIONS

It is important for the psychiatrist in the general ward to be aware of interactions between the psychotropic drugs he prescribes and other drugs. The British National Formulary has a fairly comprehensive list. Table 13.1 lists important interactions with drugs likely to be prescribed by psychiatrists.

DYING PATIENTS AND BEREAVEMENT REACTIONS

Dying patients

It is usually neither necessary nor appropriate to refer dying patients to psychiatrists. Occasionally their level of distress will be such that either they themselves or their doctors will request a consultation. Sometimes the request comes from the nursing staff or even the relatives.

In dealing with dying patients the doctor's own defence mechanisms are often quickly brought into operation. He may be confronted with fears that he won't cope and recall medical school dictums about not getting 'over-involved' with patients. This may result in inappropriate behaviours including:

— Avoidance:

Table 13.1 Interactions with drugs commonly used in psychiatry

Psychiatric drug	Interacting drug	Effect
Tricyclic antidepressant	Alcohol	Potentiation of sedating effect
	Oral contraceptives	Decreased effect of tricyclics
	Phenothiazines	Increase of tricyclic side-effects
	Disulfiram	Increased antabuse effect with alcohol
	Cimetidine	Potentiation of tricyclic effects
	Bethanidine/debrisoquine, guanethidine, clonidine	Antagonism of antihypertensive effect
	Adrenaline/noradrenaline	Potentiation of actions of adrenaline/noradrenaline
Monoamine-oxidase inhibitors (MAOIs)	Sympathomimetic amines	Hypertensive crises
	Narcotic analgesics (especially pethidine), reserpine, tricyclic antidepressants, tetrabenazine	CNS excitation and hypertension
	Antidiabetic drugs (insulin and oral hypoglycaemics)	Potentiation of antidiabetic effects
Benzodiazepine	Alcohol/tricyclies/narcotic analgesics, cimetidine, disulfiram	Potentiation of benzodiazepine effects
	L-Dopa	Occasional anatagonism of L-dopa's action
Phenothiazines	Antacids	Reduced absorption of phenothiazines
	Beta-blockers	Increased plasma concentration of phenothiazines
	Metirosine, metaclopramide	Increase extrapyramidal side-effects
Haloperidol	Indomethacin	Severe drowsiness
	Metaclopramide, metirosine	Increased extrapyramidal side-effects
Lithium	Diuretics (especially thiazides)	Potentiation of lithium's actions

Table 13.1 Cont.

Psychiatric drug	Interacting drug	Effect
	Non-steroid anti-inflammatory drugs	Potentiation of lithium's actions
	Acetazolamide/aminophylline	Increased lithium excretion
	Sodium bicarbonate	Increased lithium excretion
	Haloperidol/probably also phenothiazines	Increased extrapyramidal side-effects, neurotoxicity
Anticholinergics, e.g. benztropine or orphenadrine	Tricyclic antidepressants, antihistamines, phenothiazines, disopyramide	Increased anticholinergic side-effects, urinary retention, confusional states
Beta-blockers	Verapamil/nifedipine	Hypotension, heart failure, asystole
	Cimetidine	Increased plasma concentration of beta-blocker
	Antidiabetic drugs	Potentiation of hypoglycaemic effects (with possible masking of the symptoms)
Carbamazepine	Cimetidine, dextropropoxyphene, erythromycin, isoniazid	Potentiation of carbamazepine's effects
	Steroids, oral contraceptives	Inhibition of carbamazepine's effects
	Thyroxine	Increased thyroxine metabolism
	Warfarin	Inhibition of carbamazepine's effects
	Theophylline	Decreased theophylline levels
Disulfiram	Metronidazole	Psychotic reaction
	Tricyclic antidepressants	Increased antabuse effect with alcohol
	Benzodiazepines	Potentiation of benzodiazepine effects

- Not speaking to patients
- Banishing them to side rooms
- Not dealing with emotional aspects of their care and focusing on physical aspects

— Withholding information:
  - On treatment and its side-effects
  - On the prognosis

(This is often rationalized by saying things like 'We wouldn't want to upset him'.)

— Overintrusive treatment or investigation:
  - As an attempt to deal with the doctor's feelings of helplessness or his shortcomings
  - As a way of avoiding dealing with psychological issues

— Unrealistic reassurance:
  - As a means of avoiding unpleasant truths
  - As a way of avoiding his own intense feelings

The above comments are meant to be helpful rather than critical. All of us from time to time experience the above. This is merely an indication of our humanity, not necessarily a sign that we are not interested in our patients. It does, however, help to be aware of the above mechanisms as they can interfere with optimal management of our patients. It is only fair to mention at this point that junior doctors and nurses in particular often feel constrained in what they can say and do with the patient by what their seniors wish. If this is the case, it is perfectly reasonable to encourage patients to ask questions of consultant staff and indeed to encourage consultant staff to discuss important aspects of diagnosis, management and prognosis with the patients themselves.

Many of our patients would like more information on diagnosis, management and prognosis. Some don't, but discussing this with them usually clarifies this. McGuire has described a reflective style of interview which elicits more information from patients about what they do and don't want to know (McGuire and Faulkner 1988a,b). The following are helpful in talking to dying patients:

— As much as is feasible on a ward find a quiet suitable place to talk.
— Give patients and their relatives time to talk, express their own feelings and ask their own questions.
— Don't lie to patients:

- Don't unload the whole truth in one session (the patient will forget some of it)
- Give information in small doses
- Combine verbal with written information
— Beware committing yourself to an exact prognosis. The chances of you being wrong are high.
— As well as giving negative information give positive information, e.g. regarding pain relief.
— It may be important if death is inevitable to encourage the patients and relatives to deal with final acts:
  - Making wills
  - Sorting out financial affairs
  - Healing hurts in relationships
— Always invite questions from the patient and end by asking 'Is there anything more you would like to ask me?'
— Make sure the patient realizes you are available for further discussions in the future.

The question of depressive illness is sometimes raised in relation to dying patients. It is often difficult to diagnose as many of the symptoms of their illness may be similar to depressive symptoms, e.g. sleep disturbance, weight loss. It is however important to be alert to the possibility of depressive illness and to beware of the trap of understandability, i.e. 'Who wouldn't be depressed if they had bony metastases?'. Antidepressants will improve the quality of life for those with depressive illnesses.

It is important to ask about religious beliefs. If present these can be of enormous support to someone who is dying. Occasionally others who are ambivalent in this area may wish to discuss their ambivalence with an appropriate person, e.g. priest or minister. It is however important that the doctor does not push his religious views on to the patient as this can make his ability to cope worse.

Bereavement reactions

Textbooks on emergency medicine and psychiatry often have little to say on this matter. It is important that all doctors are familiar with the range of symptoms which may be experienced in a grief reaction, and also that they are familiar with the possible complications of bereavement. For a detailed account of this the reader is referred elsewhere (Worden 1983, Parkes 1986).

In summary there are four phases to a grief reaction:

— Numbness.
— Yearning and searching — permanence of the loss often denied at this stage. Anger may be common.
— Disorganization. Problems functioning at home and work.
— Reorganization/reintegration.

In addition, Worden has described four tasks of mourning. Bearing these four tasks in mind should enable the doctor to assist his patient through a grief reaction.

— Accepting the reality of the loss. Involves accepting the loss as real and accepting its meaning for you.
— Experiencing the pain of grief. Don't collude with efforts to avoid this. Well-meaning friends and relatives (and doctors!) sometimes do. Refusal to feel may be dangerous — it may lead to later depressive illness.
— Adjustment to an environment in which the deceased is missing. This depends on what the person has lost, e.g. spouse, sexual partner, cook, gardener.
— Reinvestment of emotional energy in new relationships. Many people fail here, they feel they are 'letting down' the bereaved by making new relationships. May need encouragement and permission to do this.

Helping people to grieve means helping them through these four tasks. This will involve helping them to an awareness of the reality and meaning of the loss (do this by allowing them to talk about the details), helping them show feelings, providing practical help (they may be eligible for certain benefits), helping them withdraw emotionally, arranging longer-term support.

It is also important to be able to identify pathological grief reactions. Grief can go wrong in several ways:

— It may be prolonged. It is difficult to say 'how long is prolonged'. Patients themselves are usually aware they are not coping and that there is no progression. Grief may go on for years and may result in depressive illness or suicide. It may result in inability to return to work or make new relationships.
— It may be delayed. Grief reactions may be totally delayed, or

there may have been a brief but inadequate early reaction. Often at some later time of loss or difficulty the inhibited affect comes to the surface and causes problems.
— It may be excessive. This does not relate as much to the length as to the quality of a grief reaction. The patient may become phobic of death, and develop irrational feelings of despair and helplessness.
— It may be concealed. Parkes talks about 'affective equivalents of grief' which are really non-affective symptoms such as psychosomatic symptoms or behavioural disturbances.

Identification or suspicion of any of these problems should lead to arrangements for longer-term follow-up being made. They cannot adequately be dealt with in the short term in emergency situations.

PRACTICE POINT
It takes people longer to get over grief than most doctors or relatives believe.

14. Emergencies in geriatric psychiatry

AIMS
Assess the psychological, physical and social factors contributing to the patient's presentation.

Evaluate the appropriate options for management and make suitable arrangements for the patient's immediate health and safety.

Arrange adequate follow-up.

INTRODUCTION

Many emergencies in geriatric psychiatry can be dealt with in the same way as in younger patients. Some aspects of assessment and particular problems of diagnosis and management merit further description and these will be covered in this chapter.

ASSESSMENT (see Ch. 3)

History taking

As a matter of routine this should involve taking a history from a relative or carer as well as from the patient. In addition to a standard psychiatric history the following are particularly relevant in the elderly:

— Level of functioning before illness. Have there been any changes in this during the onset of the patient's illness? (This will include an account of previous activities, interests etc.)
— Assessment of activities of daily living:
  • Washing
  • Dressing
  • Feeding

- Mobility
- Continence
— Assessment of family/carer's involvement:
  - Who lives with the patient?
  - Who visits and how often?
  - What supports have they been offering?
  - What are they prepared to offer in the future?
— Other services involved:
  - Home help
  - Sitter service
  - Day care
  - Other hospital services
— Other problems:
  - Concurrent ill health (including blindness and deafness)
— Is the patient refusing to accept help?
  - Family feuds

Mental state examination

This is similar to the mental state examination of younger patients (see Ch. 3) but with particular emphasis on assessment of cognitive functioning which will include:

— Alertness.
— Orientation (time, place and person).
— Speech. Any evidence of dysphasias.
— Memory:
  - Consistency of the history
  - Remembering doctor's name
  - Address after 5 minutes
  - Remembering items in a list
  - Knowledge of recent current affairs
  - Babcock sentence (a test of logical memory)
— Parietal lobe function:
  - Visuo-spacial difficulties, e.g. topographical disorientation or block copying
  - Dysphasias
  - Apraxia
  - Gerstmann's syndrome (finger agnosia, discalculia, right/left disorientation and agraphia)
  - Body image disturbance
  - Astereognosis

Physical examination

This is not always carried out in younger patients presenting as emergencies to psychiatrists. There is a particularly strong correlation between physical and mental illness in the elderly and sometimes difficulty in differential diagnosis between physical and psychiatric illness.

PRACTICE POINT
In the elderly physical examination should always be performed.

Difficulties

Difficulties in obtaining a history and examining mental state are too readily attributed to dementia by doctors. They may be due to:

— Deafness.
— Dysphasias.
— Confusion caused by other conditions (see Ch. 13).

It is important that the doctor is patient and perseveres in his efforts to assess the patient thoroughly.

Aids to communication may be helpful and include:

— Hearing aids.
— Communicators.
— Using the written word rather than the spoken word.
— Using pictures.

Relatives are often able and willing to assist. The interviewer should repeatedly reorientate the confused elderly patient to what is happening, explaining procedures clearly and simply.

ACUTE CONFUSIONAL STATES IN THE ELDERLY

The symptoms, signs, causes and management of acute confusional states have been dealt with at length in Chapter 13. We make no apology for returning to this topic here. Acute confusional states occur in 30–50% of hospitalised patients over 65 years old. They are associated with considerable morbidity and mortality and are frequently misdiagnosed. The commonest misdiagnosis is dementia, although they are occasionally mistaken for functional psychoses when mood disturbance, hallucinations or delusions appear to predominate. The

Table 14.1 Differentiation of acute confusional states from dementia

Feature	Acute confusional state	Dementia
Onset	Rapid, hours to days	Slowly progressive
Conscious level	Diminished awareness, fluctuating, poor attention	Clear conscious level though disorientated
Sleep	Disturbed, virtually always worse at night	Normal duration (for age) but sleep reversal may occur
Course	Irregular, fluctuates rapidly. Usually lasts days to a few weeks	Slowly progressive (occasionally more rapid, e.g. in vascular or viral dementias)
Clinical picture	Agitated, fearful often visual hallucinations, fleeting paranoid delusions, mood labile	Mood more flattened. Hallucinations less common and less frightening
Cause	Usually drugs or medical illness	Usually a slowly progressive cause, e.g. Alzheimer's, vascular disease

distinction from dementia is crucially important. Failure to make it has two important consequences:

— No search is made for underlying causes and significant but often treatable physical illness is thereby missed.
— Mislabelling as dementia leads to misplacement, e.g. in longstay wards.

Table 14.1 outlines the key factors which distinguish acute confusional states from dementia. It is perhaps worth re-emphasizing that acute confusional states last longer in the elderly when compared with the young. They can take several weeks to clear and if there is any diagnostic doubt the patient should be observed for at least 3 or 4 weeks and hidden underlying causes should be looked for before the label of dementia is attached.

Psychosocial causes of confusion

In addition to the causes of acute confusion listed in Chapter 13, an almost identical syndrome can occur in the elderly following major life events, e.g.:

— Relocation:
  • To hospital

- To a new house
- To an old folk's home
— Robbery/assault.
— Loss events, especially bereavement.

DEMENTIA

We have already spent some time discussing conditions which
may be mistaken for dementia. One of the reasons for this was
to emphasize the crucial importance of accurate diagnosis of
dementia. The psychiatrist must remember this, as misdiagnosis
can and often does lead to errors in both management and
placement which can take considerable time and effect to undo.
In addition to acute confusional states, depression especially with
retardation may be misdiagnosed as dementia. In a few cases
dementia may be caused by something which is reversible.
These include:

— Alcohol.
— Subdural haematoma.
— Endocrine disorders.
— Normal pressure hydrocephalus.
— Syphilis.
— Vitamin deficiencies.

The diagnosis of dementia should only be made on a history
of progressive impairment of cerebral functioning which is global
in its nature, i.e. including impairment of memory, abstract
thinking, judgement, personality and higher cortical functions,
e.g. aphasias and apraxias. Most definitions also now include
impairment in activities of daily living.

PRACTICE POINT
*It is wrong to see dementia as a disorder only of memory even if this
is often the most striking presenting feature.*

Crisis presentations

Ideally, early identification, assessment and appropriate
management should reduce the number of patients with
dementia presenting in crisis. For many reasons, however, crises
still occur. The main reasons for crises are contained in Table
14.2. These crises may lead to presentation of the patient to any

Table 14.2   Crises in dementia

Type of crisis	Examples
Crises of behaviour	Gas taps left on Water taps left on Lost in the street Disinhibited behaviour Shoplifting
Crises of care	Death of carer Illness of carer Relative arrives on holiday Relative goes on holiday Home help goes
Medical crises	Drug mistake/overdose Physical illness Acute confusion due to illness Strokes in multi-infarct dementia

Reproduced from Jacques (1988) with permission.

one of GPs, casualty officers, psychiatrists, social work departments and the police. The response to a crisis will often determine the future pattern of care. The doctor therefore must always retain a long-term view of the problem. His aim should be not only to manage the crisis but to begin to manage the long-term decline so as to avert further crises.

Negative attitudes to patients with dementia often prevail, especially in casualty departments where they are often seen as an unwanted and time-consuming intrusion into places more geared to managing acute medical emergencies. This is unfortunate as virtually all patients with dementia can be helped both in terms of their own quality of life and in terms of assisting those caring for them.

Emergency management of dementia

PRACTICE POINT
Even in emergencies it is important to remember that the management of the multiple problems of the dementia sufferer must be multidisciplinary. Those who may be involved in management include:

— General practitioner.
— Psychiatrist.
— Relatives.
— Social workers.

— Home care organizers.
— Community psychiatric nurses.
— Occupational therapists.

Knowing what services are available is the essence of good management. The psychiatrist responsible for geriatric services should ensure that those likely to have regular contact with dementia patients are informed about the services. In a good service, a psychogeriatrician will be on call 24 hours a day and the doctors faced with the emergency should not hesitate to discuss the immediate management with him.

Immediate management is heavily dependent on the situation in which the problem presents as well as on the kind of problem. For example, the management of a behaviourally disturbed patient with Alzheimer's disease who is in a general medical ward is obviously quite different to the management of a demented old man at home whose wife has just died.

Example

Only a few general principles of management can be outlined here. In Table 14.3 management of particular problems is

Table 14.3   Management of problems in dementia

Problem	Management plan
Behavioural disturbance, e.g. wandering, aggression, shouting, etc.	1. Look for underlying cause 2. Look at *where* the behaviour occurs — circumstances, environment, etc. 3. Reinforce desired behaviours — reward them 4. Treat cause/change environment if possible 5. Drugs — but think of this only after trying 1–4
Withdrawal of support, e.g. loss of spouse, family on holiday	Look at means of replacing this, e.g. increase home help, community nurse support, volunteer visitors, day centre, day hospital, before thinking of removing the patient from familiar surroundings
Intercurrent medical illness	Depending on severity of the illness and behaviour, admission may be needed. With good medical support plus the agencies mentioned above, it may be possible to help the patient at home

discussed. An example of this style of management would be to look at the problem of an 80-year-old lady with Alzheimer's disease brought to her GP because she was wandering from home and getting lost. She was frequently brought back by the police or neighbours. The approach should be as follows. Ask:

— Why does she wander? There are many possible reasons:
  • Disorientation
  • She needs exercise
  • She may want to get back home, e.g. patients wandering out of day hospitals or wards
  • She may be in pain and therefore be restless and agitated
  • It may be drug induced, e.g. akathisia
  • Anxiety
— Where and when does she wander?
  • Only from home?
  • Only from hospital ..or both?
  • Only at night?

This kind of analysis will suggest ways of treating or lessening the problem.

Table 14.4 Ways of keeping dementia sufferers in the community

Facility	Examples
1. Medical/nursing facilities	District nurse Incontinence/bathing/night nursing services Health visitor Community psychiatric nurse Day hospital/respite beds
2. Social work department	Home help Occupational therapy assessment, provision of aids Day centres Social workers — help re finance, housing, residential homes
3. Voluntary agencies — often Alzheimer's Disease Society or Age Concern	Meals on wheels Sitting services (volunteer will sit with patient for a few hours day or night) Day centres Support groups for relatives
4. Private sector	Private home helps Private sitters/nurse

Alternatives to inpatient management

In Table 14.4 some alternatives to hospitalization (often the easy option, not always the best one) are outlined. We suggest you think about all of these before admitting a patient unless his medical condition or unavailability of these services dictate otherwise.

There is much variation between local facilities so the list in Table 14.4 is merely a guide to the kinds of service which are available and which can make the difference between good community care and long stay admission. Patients with dementia do sometimes need to be admitted to hospital but this should be done only when there is a clear medical or psychiatric indication and not as an easy option. Admitting patients because 'she has to go somewhere' or 'something must be done' merely passes the problem to someone else and is neither good practice nor likely to be helpful to the patient.

We have emphasized managing the patient in crisis but in the case of dementia it is often appropriate to ask 'Who is the patient? Who is in crisis?'. The patient may not have changed but the attitude, health, or availability of a carer may have. It may be the carer to whom more support has to be directed.

15. Psychiatric emergencies in primary care

AIMS
Appreciate the range of emergencies presenting in primary care and the problems faced by GPs trying to manage those problems at home.

INTRODUCTION

It is GPs, not psychiatrists, who deal with the vast majority of psychiatric patients. About 90% of people experiencing psychiatric symptoms consult their GP. The GP will treat most of these himself, only seeking specialist help with 7% of cases (see Table 15.1).

Table 15.1 The pathway to psychiatric care

The community	Primary medical care			Specialist psychiatric care	
Population	Psychiatric morbidity in random community samples	Total psychiatric morbidity attending GP	Psychiatric morbidity identified by GP	Total psychiatric patients	Psychiatric inpatients
1000 →	250 →	230 →	140 →	17 →	6
		(per thousand population at risk per year)			

Adapted from Goldberg and Huxley (1980) with permission.

EPIDEMIOLOGY

The GP will also be seeing a very different range of psychiatric disorders, both in diagnosis and severity, compared with the psychiatrist. It has been calculated that the average general practice with a list of 2500 patients will contain:

— 5 known and 25 unknown cases of chronic alcoholism.
— 5–10 problem families.
— 60 one-parent families.
— 12 cases of severe depression.
— 3 parasuicides (one suicide every 3 years).
— 55 chronically mentally ill.
— 10 mentally handicapped people.
— 300 neurotic disorders.

The major diference between psychiatric emergencies
presenting to the GP and those seen by psychiatrists (even those
who refer themselves to psychiatrists) is the presence of physical
symptoms, fear of physical illness, and true physical illness
complicating the presentation. The 'hidden psychiatric
morbidity', those patients with psychiatric symptoms that are
missed by the GP (see Table 15.1), are nearly all diagnosed as
suffering from minor physical conditions.

EMERGENCIES PRESENTING IN GENERAL PRACTICE

Common emergencies

— Anxiety with panic attacks.
— Domestic crises including violence.
— 'Reactive' depression.
— Alcohol problems.
— Breavement reactions.
— Confusion in the elderly.

Less common emergencies

— Self-harm.
— Drug abuse:
  • Demands for drugs
— Major psychoses:
  • Severe depression
  • Schizophrenia

Complicating factors

— Demand for immediate relief of symptoms.
— Demand for medication.
— Alcohol.

ASSESSMENT BY GENERAL PRACTITIONERS

Psychiatric emergencies may be seen in the surgery, in the patient's home or occasionally elsewhere. GPs are contracted to provide emergency care for anyone who happens to become ill within the practice catchment area. Most commonly in Britain this will involve a home visit which can produce specific difficulties. For example, it may be a relative, neighbour, friend or the patient who opens the door. It can be very embarrassing to find that you are assessing the wrong person!

The assessment will be similar to that described in Chapter 3 but the following points should be borne in mind by the GP:

— Ask the name and relationship of each person present.
— Try to see the patient as soon as possible, particularly if he is distressed or suspicious. He may feel that you will be biased by persuasive relatives.
— Ask the patient whether he wants to be seen alone or with someone else present except where there is a risk of violence (see Ch. 9).
— The assessment needs to be focused (see Ch. 3).

Assessing a patient at home can be much more difficult than assessing the same patient in the security of the hospital. The patient may be less cooperative, the relatives may be exerting pressure on the doctor and the GP may feel threatened.

DOMICILIARY ASSESSMENT BY PSYCHIATRISTS

Most domiciliary assessments will be carried out by consultants or senior registrars, but in some services this task is delegated to more junior trainees who may be teamed up with a more senior colleague from another discipline.

PRACTICE POINT
Do not fall into the trap of criticizing the GP's request for a second opinion or admission. It is difficult to assess and manage many patients at home without the support of a a psychiatric team or specialist training.

If in doubt about the reason for the referral, telephone the GP for further information.

Patients seen by psychiatrists at home are amongst the most severely ill or disabled of the patients they encounter. They are

very different from the majority of emergencies seen and
managed by the GP. It is often helpful to invite the GP to
introduce you to the patient. This also means that the GP will
be available to give you additional information and discuss your
findings and management plan.

Problems

The domiciliary visit is not always as easy as one might think.
The following should be considered:

— What if the patient refuses to open the door? Particularly
  where the patient is paranoid, he may be frightened of
  letting a stranger into the house:
  • Do not give up immediately. If you fail to see the patient
    the problem will not just go away
  • It is possible to conduct a reasonable assessment by
    speaking through the letter box!
  • You may then be able to persuade the patient to let you
    in or decide whether there are grounds for admission
    under the Mental Health Act
  • If there is no answer at all contact the GP. You will need
    to discuss whether there is any particular cause for alarm.
    The GP may decide to contact the police
— Remember violence (see Ch. 9):
  • You are walking into an unknown situation when you
    enter a patient's house
  • Be on your guard and assess the risks involved
  • If in doubt, leave and arrange to return with a colleague
— Transport to hospital:
  • Do not attempt to drive a patient to hospital in your car,
    especially if on your own
  • This could be hazardous (if the patient became agitated
    and distracted you, or attempted to leave the car) and
    you may be uninsured
  • Always arrange for relatives or the ambulance service to
    transport patients
— Inform someone of your movements:
  • For your own safety ensure that someone knows your
    timetable — who you are going to see, where and
    approximately when

- If you do get into difficulty then that person (your secretary in most cases) can alert others if you fail to make contact in a reasonable time

This section has focused on problems. In fact, domiciliary assessment and treatment can be extremely interesting and rewarding.

16. Referrals from the police

AIMS
Collect sufficient information to provide a psychiatric assessment.
Conduct the examination in a proper setting.
Liaise with local psychiatric services.

INTRODUCTION

The police are a regular source of referrals to any psychiatric emergency service. The actual process of referral, however, varies considerably over the UK. In many cases the police will simply direct people in distress to local psychiatric services. Mental health legislation also authorizes a police constable who finds a person who appears to be suffering from mental disorder in a place to which the public has access, to remove him to a 'place of safety'. A place of safety may be a hospital or a police station and which is prefered varies considerably across the UK. In some parts of the country senior trainees provide a psychiatric emergency service to the police to assess people in custody. Such a service may also be offered by police surgeons who have had special experience in psychiatry. Although these regional variations mean that few generalizations can be made, we felt it was important to include this chapter because of certain difficulties that complicate the assessment of referrals from the police.

REASONS FOR REFERRAL

The reasons for referral are broadly similar to those encountered in emergency psychiatric clinics or in a busy casualty department. However, it is more likely you will be asked to see someone who is disturbed in his behaviour, rather than someone who is withdrawn and depressed. The most common reasons for referral are:

— Threat of self-harm, e.g. jumping from a height, and then taken to a place of safety, either a police station or a hospital, to be assessed by a medical practitioner.
— Actual self-harm.
— Bizarre or eccentric behaviour, e.g. wandering naked, talking to imaginary companions.
— People in custody (if a service is provided to police stations) who are:
  • At high risk of self-harm, e.g. banging head against cell wall
  • Known to have received psychiatric treatment, particularly if associated with any of the above features

ASSESSMENT

Steps in the assessment of a person referred by the police are:

— Clarify what you are asked to do, e.g. determine whether it is safe for a person to remain in police custody.

PRACTICE POINT
Do not attempt to determine fitness to plead, nor issues of criminal responsibility as an emergency. Such requests are not urgent matters and should be redirected to the psychiatric forensic service.

— Determine the circumstances of arrest — not always proferred. The police are not necessarily familiar with how psychiatrists conduct an examination. You may find the police keen to usher you straight to see the person. It is important that you gather the following information:
  • How did the police become involved?
  • What was the person's behaviour at the time?
  • How did the person explain this behaviour?
  • Has the person's appearance changed, e.g. a naked person been clothed, or bizarre item of clothing removed?
  • Was an offence committed?
  • What is the legal status of the person, e.g. removed to a place of safety, arrested or charged.
    Unfortunately the policeman who first detains the person may not be present; however, it is likely that he will be contactable

by telephone or by radio. This is particularly relevant where
someone has been detained after an attempt at self-harm (see
below).
— Collect existing information about the person. Never neglect
sources of information other than the police and the person
himself. For example, the person may have hospital records
or a key worker. Other sources of information are given in
Chapter 2.
— Decide if it is appropriate to see the person alone.

PRACTICE POINT
*It is particularly important in forensic psychiatry to ask yourself
whether it is appropriate to see the person alone (see Chs 2 and 9).*

— If necessary, insist on a proper setting for the examination.
You may be asked to examine someone at a police station. A
police cell may be cramped or unhygienic. Insist on a
properly equipped interview room where you may have a
confidential interview (see Ch. 2).
— Examine the patient. There is nothing extraordinary about
the history or mental state examination in such circumstances
(see Ch. 3). Despite any misgivings, you will probably find
that you are confronted with a common clinical problem.

Suicide risk

The assessment of a person who has threatened self-harm is a
common clinical problem in such referrals. The guidelines for
the assessment of suicidal intent have already been covered in
Chapter 6. However, this is a good example of an occasion when
it is necessary to obtain detailed information about the
circumstances of how the person came into contact with the
police. There is a great difference in suicidal intent between
someone found by chance in the dead of night sitting in a car
on an isolated country road with a hosepipe attached the exhaust
pipe, and someone running in front of cars in a busy town
centre. The police might consider both to be equally at risk of
suicide.

MANAGEMENT

The principles of emergency management have already been
given in Chapter 4. A few points, however, merit special emphasis.

The decision to charge

The police may bring a person who has displayed disturbed behaviour voluntarily to an emergency psychiatric clinic. You may learn while collecting information about the person that if you do not admit him to hospital, then he will be taken to a police station and charged with an offence. Consequently, you may feel under pressure to manage the person in a certain way. However, such pressure should be consciously ignored in your management plan.

Fitness to remain in custody

There will be few occasions when a person is so ill that they are not safe in police custody. Examples are:

— Acute florid psychosis:
  • Schizophrenic excitement
  • Manic excitement
  • Depressive stupor
— Acute confusional states.
— Several alcohol withdrawal, e.g. delirium tremens (see Appendix 2: case history 12).

Drug treatment

Occasionally there will be times when you feel it would be appropriate to prescribe a psychotropic drug to a person in police custody, e.g. a benzodiazepine to someone suffering mild to moderate alcohol withdrawal symptoms. On the one hand, such treatment may make both the person and the police feel better; however, who will administer and supervise the drug treatment once you have left? In most cases administering a drug without proper supervision is best avoided. In some parts of the country, such supervision may be offered by a police surgeon.

LIAISON WITH LOCAL SERVICES

In the organization of an emergency psychiatric service, it is important to know:

— Where persons who appear to be suffering from mental disorder will be taken by the police for psychiatric

assessment, e.g. police station, casualty department or local psychiatric hospital?
— Whether a service will be provided to the police for assessment of persons in custody.
— If such services are to be organized, who will be responsible, e.g. the forensic or general adult service?
— The role of local police surgeons.

17. Crisis intervention

AIMS
See the patient as part of a family or social system which is in difficulty.
Help the whole system cope more effectively.

INTRODUCTION

Much confusion surrounds the term *crisis intervention*. It has been applied (or rather, misapplied) to a range of services provided by volunteers and professionals, from telephone befriending services (e.g. Samaritans) to conventional acute psychiatric services offering short-stay hospital admission. In Britain it is frequently used as a synonym for emergency home visiting and treatment teams. In fact every psychiatrist should be able to use the techniques of crisis intervention. These are skills to be used selectively with individuals who are not ill but in *crisis*. It provides a framework for dealing immediately and vigorously with a patient's acute reactions to overwhelming life-events. It therefore depends on an understanding of *normal coping mechanisms* and how to facilitate problem-solving.

THEORY

The normal coping process

This was first described in relation to bereavement:

— Stage 1. Immediate response:
  - Numbness
  - Disbelief
— Stage 2. Full reaction:
  - Anxiety

- Distress
- Anger
- Guilt
- Regression
- Inertia
- Depression
— Stage 3. Resolution:
  - Acceptance and planning for the future

It is recognized now that the coping process is used in a variety of events including:

Loss

— Bereavement.
— Break up of relationships or marriage.
— Loss of job.
— Loss of expectations, e.g.:
  - Not being promoted
  - Failing exam
  - Miscarriage
  - Birth of handicapped child

Change

— Developmental:
  - Adolescence
  - Having children
  - Menopause
  - Failing health in old age
— Relationships:
  - Leaving home
  - Marriage
  - Children leaving home
— Career:
  - Leaving school
  - Starting at college or work
  - Graduation or promotion

PRACTICE POINT
Desirable life changes such as marriage or promotion at work, may provoke crisis.

These changes produce a new set of responsibilities, relationships and, importantly, may alter the support available.

Model of crisis

Why is it that some people cope with these stresses while others fail and are precipitated into crisis? Caplan has suggested the following useful model, shown in Figure 17.1.

Caplan suggests that each person is in a state of *emotional equilibrium* which is regularly upset by threats. Most of these are minor, causing a brief and frequently undetectable rise in tension (Stage 1) which automatically sparks off coping responses which deal with the problem and restore emotional equilibrium.

Example. Walking into a social gathering late, I might quite automatically crack a joke at my own expense, defusing the situation.

If the threat is greater, these automatic responses fail to work and there is a further rise in tension which is now felt as

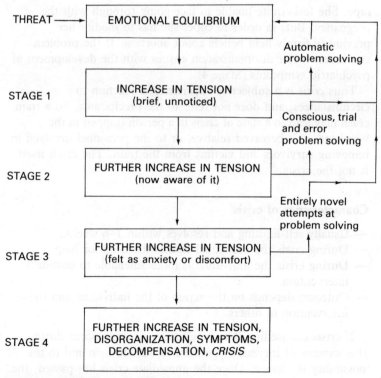

Figure 17.1 Caplan's model of crisis

discomfort or anxiety (Stage 2). Conscious attempts are now made to resolve the problem. These may be disorganized, trial and error attempts.

Example. Having been caught shoplifting an individual might, in quick succession:

— Deny the charge.
— Try to pay for the goods.
— Admit the charge but try to claim amnesia.
— Admit the charge and ask to contact a lawyer.

Faced with a major threat which has not been resolved by Stage 2 mechanisms, there is a further rise in tension which mobilizes completely new ways of coping (Stage 3). The individual's firmly held beliefs may be challenged, or the problem may have to be redefined so that only part of it is tackled.

Example. A young woman who is an active member of an anti-abortion organization finds that she is pregnant following a rape. She feels quite unable to face going through with the pregnancy. But, in order to cope, she has to modify her previously firmly held beliefs about abortion. If the problem continues, major disorganization ensues with the development of psychiatric symptoms (Stage 4).

Thus *crisis* is a subjective experience, a reaction to circumstances, and does not refer to the precipitants. So a train crash may lead to a state of crisis in a person trapped in the wreckage, to a bereaved relative, or to the personnel involved in removing survivors and victims from the train. The crash itself is not the crisis.

Characteristics of crisis

— Usually self-limiting and resolves within 1–6 weeks.
— During crisis the individual signals the need for help.
— During crisis the individual is more amenable to outside intervention.
— Outcome depends on the action of the individual and the intervention of others.

If crisis counselling is to be effective, it must occur during this window of increased openness to outside help and to the possibility of change. Once the immediate crisis has passed, the situation becomes 'fossilized' and motivation and capacity to change is diminished. But since nothing has been resolved, it is inevitable that tensions will again rise in due course and a further opportunity for intervention will occur.

Characteristics of crisis intervention

Crisis intervention involves offering appropriate help to:

— Facilitate communication.
— Enable an accurate appraisal of the problem.
— Help with the appropriate expression of feelings.
— Bolster self-esteem.
— Mobilize support.
— Promote effective problem solving.

It is:

— Time limited.
— Involves not just the individual, but his family.
— Problem orientated.
— Promotes self-reliance rather than dependence.
— Treats the individual as someone with problems rather than illness.

THE CRISIS INTERVIEW

The crisis interview has much in common with the normal emergency assessment described in Chapter 3.

PRACTICE POINT
A crisis interview is both an assessment and therapeutic session combined.

How to start the interview

— Introduce yourself and any other professional person present.
— Identify family members and their relationship to the patient.
— Tell what you know already.
— From the outset make it clear that the whole family will have a role to play in resolving the crisis.

What to ask first

— The main problems:
  • Symptoms

- ● Coping
- ● Practical
— Focus on the previous 2–3 weeks, especially life changes or events.
— Incorporate a mental state examination into the session by collecting information throughout. For example, it is less disruptive to note ability to concentrate on questions and discussion rather than asking 'serial sevens'. Similarly, orientation and memory can be assessed surreptitiously.
— Any previous psychiatric contact.

Involve family and facilitate communication

— Generate a problem list from the family group.
— Ensure that everyone is involved.
— Be a good role model, e.g. show that you are listening to what each person is saying.

PRACTICE POINT
Relatives often devalue the patient's point of view once they have decided that he is ill. It is vital that you demonstrate that you are treating his point of view as seriously as those of his relatives.

Accurate appraisal followed by a contract

— Give the family your appraisal of the situation. Make a connection between the symptoms of crisis and the problem list, i.e. the crisis is understandable.
— Discuss the advantages and disadvantages of:
  - ● Hospital admission
  - ● Day hospital
  - ● Support at home

If there is difficulty in coping rather than illness, it is better to deal with the problems at home rather than insulated from them in hospital.

— Offer a contract:
  - ● Explain the commitments on both sides
  - ● Agree to see the family regularly over a fixed period of time (3–6 weeks)
  - ● Agree that the whole family including the patient will work to resolve the problem

Using the problem list for planning

Problems faced by the family or system may be:

— Insoluble in the short term:
  - Ignore
— Potentially soluble:
  - Make these the focus of discussion

In planning the intervention:

— Focus family resources on solving the problems about which something can be done.
— Explore different solutions.
— Allocate tasks.
— Identify and mobilize supports.
— Arrange support for the therapist (see Ch. 18).

PRACTICAL EXAMPLE

George, a 30-year-old married man, was referred to the duty psychiatrist by his GP because of 'profound suicidal depression requiring immediate hospital admission'. He arrived at the hospital outpatient department with his wife and young baby. He was interviewed by the duty registrar and a student social worker.

Start of interview

The following statements could be made by either member of the crisis team. Both should take an equal part.

'My name is Dr A. I am the duty psychiatrist. This is Ms B who is a social work student working with the emergency team'.
'Can we just be clear who you are?' (Let them introduce themselves.)
'Your GP phoned to let us know that you would be coming. He told us that you had become depressed and had been thinking about ending your life. He wondered if you ought to be in hospital.'
'This is obviously a situation that is affecting both of you, and it will be important for both of you to be involved in any plan to try and sort out this problem.'

Initial information

— Felt 'depressed' and unable to cope for past week. Not getting out of bed, not helping in the house. A week ago

hoped he would not wake in morning. Difficulty coping with severe progressive deafness.
— Distressed but not clinically depressed. No biological symptoms of depression. No suicidal plans.
— Unable to work since a 'nervous breakdown' 3 years ago. Requesting readmission.

Wife involved

A catalogue of problems were collected from George and his wife:

— His mother, a very dominant woman, was on a month's visit from Australia. George could not cope with her, nor could he ask her to leave.
— His wife had given birth to their fourth child only a week ago.
— A further ear operation was imminent.
— The parish priest, from whom he gained a great deal of support, was on holiday for a week.
— Financial problems connected with continued unemployment.

Appraisal and contract

The couple were told that this was difficulty coping with a series of major stresses rather than illness.

— Hospital admission, while making George feel better in the short term, would solve nothing. These were problems that had to be tackled.
— The crisis could be expected to resolve in a few weeks.
— In return for regular support and help over the next month, the couple agreed to carry out the plans worked out in the sessions.

Note that hospital admission was not refused. The clear message was given that the therapists thought the couple would cope, but if they did not, then hospital admission would be arranged.

Problem list and planning

— The immediate precipitants of the crisis were the simultaneous arrival of George's mother and new baby.

— His usual supports were reduced:
  • Priest was on holiday
  • Wife's attention was taken up by needs of the baby
— Unresolved feelings surrounding mother did not allow George to ask her to leave.
— Longstanding financial problems and the operation could not be tackled immediately.
— It was acknowledged that the only solution, as George saw it, was to retire from the scene and seek asylum in hospital.
— With support George and his wife were able to share some of their anxieties with each other and both were encouraged to show their feelings e.g. not only was George allowed to cry, but his wife also.
— They were helped to discuss their problems with his mother. As the therapists predicted, George's mother did not take offence when George suggested that she might spend the next week with his sister nearby to allow the couple to get used to the new baby.
— The health visitor was asked to provide additional support for George's wife.
— Regular contact with the crisis team was offered until the priest returned.

The psychiatric team withdrew after three closely spaced visits.

18. Supervision and support

AIMS
Ensure that emergency work is a learning experience.
Do not hesitate to ask for adequate supervision.

INTRODUCTION

Emergency work is difficult and stressful. You should not be expected to be capable of making expert assessments and giving specialist advice until you have had time to gain that knowledge and expertise. Therefore, for some time you will need access to good quality supervision and support. With time and experience this need declines, but throughout your training appropriate supervision should be available.

PREPARATION FOR BEING ON CALL

— Find out who your immediate senior is and how he may be contacted.
— It may help to make contact with the senior 'on call' in order to:
  • Introduce yourself (particularly if you are in a large training scheme)
  • Inform your supervisor of your level of experience (or inexperience) and therefore the support you require
  • Find out when your supervisor wants to be contacted
  • Set up a meeting during normal working hours to discuss the cases you have managed.

PRACTICE POINT
It pays to plan ahead. Know who to contact and where before an emergency arises.

157

— Make sure you know where you can find practical
information:
  • Is there a doctors' handbook?
  • What are the catchment areas of the hospital and the
    individual admission units?
  • Guidelines for admission to appropriate inpatient unit (see
    Ch. 5)
— Consultants who, after all, ultimately carry the responsibility
  for decisions about patients you see on their behalf, often
  like to be involved in decision making. They would rather be
  called *before* the decision has been carried out rather than
  merely being informed of what has happened after the event.

WHEN TO TELEPHONE

This will depend on your level of experience and the prevailing
culture of the service. As a rule of thumb the following might
be useful:

— During your first few months you should discuss all
  emergencies seen and should expect a senior to see and
  assess particularly difficult cases.
— With experience you should discuss difficult cases,
  particularly those where you are considering hospital
  admission for the first time, but should still request a senior
  to assess the most difficult cases.
— Do not put off telephoning until a crisis occurs. Alert the
  senior early if you anticipate problems.
— If you are not coping, let someone know. It is not a sign of
  failure, incompetence or uncertainty. Trainees are respected
  if they recognize their level of competence and do not
  attempt to deal with problems that are outside their level of
  training or experience. Remember the patient must come
  first, not your pride.
— Do not give 'expert' advice to others unless you are certain
  of your knowledge. It is better to refer telephone calls from
  GPs, social workers or the police to the senior registrar or
  consultant on call (see Ch. 1).

FEEDBACK

In many services 'on call' is seen as a piece of work to be done,
and the sooner it is over and forgotten about the better.

Although you might tend to agree with these sentiments, making emergency assessments is an important part of training. You will only benefit from the experience if you have the opportunity to discuss the patients you assess and the decisions you make. This requires regular feedback.

Models of feedback

Review during a spell on duty

The supervising psychiatrist (senior registrar or consultant) comes into the hospital during the evening to discuss the patients seen so far. A less satisfactory alternative is to have a telephone review.

Debriefing session

A face-to-face meeting between the trainee and the supervising psychiatrist at the end of the spell on call to review all cases assessed and decisions made. There should be time to discuss differential diagnoses and alternative ways of handling difficult situations.

Group feedback

A less regular meeting where a number of trainees present patients they assessed for group comment. The group could be taken by a consultant or a senior trainee.

Written feedback

What does happen to patients you admit to another part of the hospital? Some hospitals arrange to send a copy of discharge summaries to the emergency doctor responsible for the admission. If you have no opportunity to discuss your emergency work except when you have a particular problem, you might want to think about what sort of feedback discussion would be appropriate and realistic for your service.

SUPPORT

Any 'on call' work is stressful. Even when nothing is happening it is difficult to relax as, at any moment, you might be called on to tackle a serious problem. Often the situation is compounded by lack of sleep and physical tiredness. You will often be asked to make decisions that, during normal working hours would be made by someone much more senior and experienced. Your responsibilities on call may extend to parts of the hospital that you hardly knew existed. Out of hours your normal supports, the other trainees and familiar colleagues are not around. So not only is the job difficult but the people to whom you normally turn are not available.

Models of support

— Regular support:
- Trainees' support group (peer group)
- Individual supervision or support (consultant or SR)
- Informally — other members of the team
— Special support:
- After any incident (violence, threats, suicide, etc.) there should be the opportunity to ventilate feelings about the experience. This may be at a debriefing session, special meeting with your consultant, or some other local arrangement

The 'regular support' should be available to all trainees, but it might not always be formally arranged. Thus, the peer group support might well consist of informal discussion over lunch or before a day-release training course. In other centres formal meetings will be part of the programme. 'Special support' after incidents is much less common. Trainees may wish to take the initiative by suggesting such a system.

References and Suggested Reading

Chapters 1-5

Bancroft J 1979 Crisis intervention. In: Bloch S (ed) An introduction to the psychotherapies. Oxford University Press, Oxford

Departments of Psychiatry and Child Psychiatry: Institute of Psychiatry and the Maudsley Hospital London 1987 Psychiatric examination. Notes on eliciting and recording clinical information in psychiatric patients, 2nd edn. Oxford Medical Publications, Oxford

Leff J P, Isaacs A D 1978 Psychiatric examination in clinical practice. Blackwell Scientific, Oxford

Lishman W A 1987 Organic psychiatry, 2nd edn. Blackwell Scientific, Oxford

Loudon J B 1988 Drug treatments. In: Kendell R E, Zealley A K (eds) Companion to psychiatric studies, 4th edn. Churchill Livingstone, Edinburgh

Pullen I M, Yellowless A J 1985 Is communication improving between general practitioners and psychiatrists? British Medical Journal 290: 31-33

Silverstone T, Turner P 1988 Drug treatment in psychiatry, 4th edn. Routledge and Kegan Paul, London

Sims A C P 1988 Symptoms in the mind. Ballière-Tindall, London

Chapter 6

Beck A T, Schuyler D, Herman I 1974 In: Beck A T, Besnick H C P, Lettien D J (eds) The prediction of suicide. Charles Press, New York

Beck A T, Steer R A, Kovacs M, Garrison B 1985 Hopelessness and eventual suicide: a 10 year prospective study of patients hospitalised with suicidal ideation. American Journal of Psychiatry 142: 559-563

Goldberg R J 1987 The use of constant observation with potentially suicidal patients in general hospitals. Hospital and Community Psychiatry 38: 303-305

Hawton K, Catalan J 1987 Attempted suicide. A practical guide to its nature and management, 2nd edn. Oxford Medical Publications, Oxford

Chapter 7

Ritson B 1986 Recognition and treatment of alcohol-related disorders. *The Practitioner* 230: 435-441

Chapter 8
Controlled Drugs and Drug Dependence 1989 In: British National
    Formulary British Medical Association and Royal Pharmaceutical
    Society of Great Britain, London
Renton T W 1987 AIDS related psychiatric disorder. British Journal of
    Psychiatry 151: 579–588
Miller D 1987 Living with AIDS and HIV. Macmillan Education,
    London
Plant M A 1987 Drugs in perspective. Hodder and Stoughton, London
Chapter 10
Departments of Psychiatry and Child Psychiatry: Institute of Psychiatry
    and the Maudsley Hospital London 1987 Op cit.
McGrath G, Bowker M 1987 Common psychiatric emergencies. Wright,
    Guildford
Murphy G E, Guze S B 1963 Setting limits: the management of the
    manipulative patient. American Journal of Psychotherapy 14: 30–47
Sims A C P 1988 Op cit.
Chapter 11
American Psychiatric Association 1987 Diagnostic and statistical manual
    of mental disorders, 3rd edn revised. Washington, American
    Psychiatric Association.
City of Bradford Metropolitan Council 1986 Out of the valley: Bradford
    MDCs response to the Bradford City Fire Disaster 1985–86
Department of Health and Social Security 1988 Diagnosis of child
    sexual abuse: guidance for doctors. HMSO, London
Ettedgui E, Bridges M 1985 Post traumatic stress disorder. Psychiatric
    Clinics of North America 8: 89–103
Chapter 12
Gershon S, Bassuk E 1980 Psychiatric emergencies: an overview.
    American Journal of Psychiatry 137: 1–11
Waldron G 1982 Psychiatric emergencies. In: Creed F, Pfeffer J M
    (eds) Medicine and psychiatry: a practical approach. Pitman, London
Chapter 13
British National Formulary. Op cit.
Creed F 1985 Life events and physical illness. Journal of Psychosomatic
    Research 29: 113–123
Ford C V 1983 The somatizing disorders: illness as a way of life.
    Elsevier Biomedical, New York
Kellner R 1986 Somatization and hypochondriasis. Praeger, New York
Lipowski Z J 1983 Transient cognitive disorders (delirium, acute
    confusional states) in the elderly. American Journal of Psychiatry
    140: 1426–1436
Maguire P, Faulkner A 1988a How to communicate with cancer
    patients: 1. Handling bad news and difficult questions. British
    Medical Journal 297: 907–909
Maguire P, Faulkner A 1988b How to communicate with cancer
    patients: 2. Handling uncertainty, collusion, and denial. British
    Medical Journal 297: 972–974
Parkes C M 1986 Bereavement, studies of grief in adult life, 2nd edn.
    Pelican, Harmondsworth

Worden W J 1983 Grief counselling and grief therapy. Tavistock, London

Chapter 14
Jacques A 1988 Understanding dementia. Churchill Livingstone, Edinburgh

Chapter 15
Goldberg D, Huxley P 1980 Mental illness in the community. Tavistock, London

Chapter 17
Aguilera D A, Messick J M 1986 Crisis intervention, theory and methodology, 5th edn. C V Mosby, St Louis
Bancroft J 1979 Crisis intervention. In: Bloch S (ed) An introduction to the psychotherapies. Oxford University Press, Oxford
Ewing C P 1978 Crisis intervention as psychotherapy. Oxford University Press, New York

Appendix 1
Use of mental health legislation in emergencies

In this section we deal only with short-term emergency holding powers and short-term emergency admission to hospital. Longer-term admission for assessment and/or treatment will not be covered. We will refer to the Mental Health (Scotland) Act 1984, the Mental Health Act 1983 (England and Wales) and the Mental Health Order (Northern Ireland) 1986. Specific indications for emergency detention are dealt with throughout the text. In this section we confine ourselves to the legal requirements for such detention. Basically throughout the UK requirements for emergency admission by a doctor are similar. Compulsory admission for assessment may be recommended if:

— The patient suffers from mental disorder AND
— It is urgently necessary for his health or safety or for the protection of other persons that he be admitted to hospital.

In Scotland, England and Wales this is all that need be said to compulsorily detain a patient. In Northern Ireland the doctor must give the grounds for his opinion that the patient suffers from mental disorder. He must spell out the evidence of that mental disorder. In all four countries the consent of relatives or a mental health officer (called an approved social worker in Northern Ireland) should be obtained. The appropriate legislation is as follows:

SCOTLAND

Outpatients

Outpatients may be detained using Section 24 of the Mental Health (Scotland) Act 1984. Detention lasts 72 hours from the time of admission. The doctor must have seen the patient on the

day on which he signs the appropriate form. This provides
authority for removal of the patient at any time within a period
of 3 days from the date on which the form was signed.

Inpatients

If the patient is already in hospital Section 25 of the Act may be
used to detain the patient. Again detention lasts 72 hours from
the time at which it was made.

If a patient on Section 24 or 25 absconds during the period of
compulsory detention he may be brought back to hospital within
this 72-hour period for which the detention order runs.
Prescribed forms for Section 24 and 25 exist and where available
these should be used. If these are unavailable it is possible to
detain the patient provided a written record is made of this
using the same wording as appears in the Mental Health Act.

ENGLAND AND WALES

Outpatients fulfilling the criteria for emergency admission may
be admitted using Section 4 of the Mental Health Act 1983
(England and Wales). This also lasts 72 hours. The patient must
be admitted within 24 hours of the doctor signing the
appropriate form. The relative or social worker consenting must
have seen the patient within the previous 24 hours. The doctor
must state that admission under Section 2 of the Act should
involve undesirable delay and if the doctor is not known to the
patient a statement explaining why admission could not have
been made by a doctor who knew the patient has to be made.

Inpatients

Inpatients can be detained using Section 5(2) of the Act. Again
the patient may be detained for up to 72 hours. This section has
to be applied by the doctor in charge of the patient's treatment.
This is usually interpreted as the consultant in charge. It does
not have to be made by a psychiatrist but where the doctor is
not a psychiatrist a senior psychiatrist should see the patient as
soon as possible in order to determine the need for further
detention.

If a patient absconds whilst detained under Section 4 or 5(2) of the Act he may be brought back to the hospital within the 72-hour period for which the detention orders run.

NORTHERN IRELAND

Outpatients

Emergency admission for assessment can be made under Article 4 of the Mental Health Order (Northern Ireland) 1986. Unlike in Scotland, England and Wales the recommendation has to be made by the patient's general practitioner or by a previously acquainted doctor. It cannot be made unless deemed urgently necessary by a doctor on the staff of the hospital to which admission is sought. The doctor making the recommendation must have seen the patient in the previous 48 hours. The patient may be taken to hospital within 48 hours of the time of the recommendation. On the day of admission the hospital doctor must see the patient and report on a prescribed form to his health board immediately. If the doctor is the responsible medical officer or a medical officer appointed by the Mental Health Commission for Northern Ireland the emergency admission can then last 7 days (this 7-day period may be extended to a 14-day period if a treatment order is to be pursued). If another hospital doctor sees the patient a period of emergency detention may last only 48 hours.

Inpatients

Inpatients may be detained under Article 7(2) of the Order. Recommendation is made by a doctor on the staff of the hospital and lasts for 48 hours.

NURSES HOLDING ORDERS

In all UK countries nurses of certain prescribed classes (in practice this means nurses trained in mental illness or mental handicap) are empowered by the mental health legislation to detain patients in hospital pending the arrival of a doctor. The conditions for this detention are the same as those conditions outlined at the beginning of this appendix for any emergency admission. The appropriate legislation is as follows:

Scotland

Patients can be held under Section 25(2) of the Mental Health (Scotland) Act 1984. The period of detention lasts 2 hours. The nurse must record in writing the time of detention and the fact that the appropriate conditions have been fulfilled. Detention ends with the arrival of a doctor who has powers to make emergency recommendations.

England and Wales

Detention may be carried out under Section 5(4) of the Mental Health (England and Wales) Act 1983. It may last for up to 6 hours. Again it ends with the arrival of a doctor empowered to recommend emergency detention. Two prescribed forms (13 and 16) must be signed and given to the hospital managers.

Northern Ireland

Detention may be carried out under Article 7(3) of the Mental Health Order 1986. Detention lasts 6 hours and ends with the arrival of a doctor who can recommend emergency detention. A prescribed form must be filled in and delivered to the responsible health board.

REPETITION OF EMERGENCY DETENTION

With reference to both emergency admission by doctors and to nurses holding powers the consecutive use of these short-term detention orders is forbidden. The precise meaning of the word 'consecutive' is not clear, but it is not within the spirit of the mental health legislation to follow up one short-term detention order immediately with another one.

Appendix 2
Case histories

Case history 1 — assessment and management: the depressed patient sent home

A 39-year-old married woman was referred by her GP to the emergency clinic at a psychiatric hospital. When she had seen her GP that morning she had burst into tears and said that she was worried that life was not worth living. She attended with her 42-year-old husband who was a joiner.

She complained that she had had to give up her part-time job as a waitress because she could not cope. She found it very difficult to meet people at work and had also stopped attending the Women's Guild because she felt so panicky. She admitted to disturbed sleep and she had no idea why she should have felt like that. Her husband was very concerned about her and told the doctor that for the past 2 weeks she had been weeping occasionally and had been very irritable with her two children. There was no family history of psychiatric illness. After the birth of her first child 12 years ago, she had been weepy for several days but had no other past psychiatric history. She was otherwise well and was receiving no treatment from her own GP.

On examination she was smartly dressed but she wore no make-up and her hair had not been done. In her talk she was self-reproachful, saying that she was letting her family and workmates down. She appeared depressed and admitted that she had thoughts that life was not worth living. However she would never have done anything to herself because of the effect this would have had on her children and husband. There were no psychotic features and her concentration was impaired.

Opinion

Depressive illness. No known precipitants.

Management

The diagnosis was explained to the couple. She was advised that she would get better although any treatment might take some time to work.

She was advised to consult her GP to receive a course of amitriptyline. The side-effects of the medicine were explained. She was sent home in the company of her husband and advised to stay off work. Her GP was telephoned and amitriptyline was recommended. She was sent a hospital outpatient appointment for 1 week later.

Case history 2 — assessment and management: the depressed patient admitted

A 68-year-old widower who was a retired bank manager was referred to the emergency clinic at a psychiatric hospital. He had lived alone in his own house since his wife died 2 years previously. He had little social life because he suffered from chronic obstructive airways disease and attended his GP regularly. That morning he had consulted his GP because he was concerned about a cough. During that interview he broke down into tears.

Over the past few weeks he had been increasingly worried about his chest. His GP had found no evidence of an exacerbation in his physical condition. He went out little but usually spent most of his time reading or doing jigsaws. Recently he had found he was unable to concentrate on either. His appetite was never good but he thought he might have lost weight recently. He had been waking early in the morning and lay worrying about his health.

There was no family history of psychiatric illness and he had no past psychiatric history. He had no financial worries and there had been no recent life events. He usually cooked for himself and looked after the house on his own. Recently he had found this more of an effort. He used a steroid inhaler regularly and occasionally required courses of antibiotics. He had given up cigarette smoking 10 years previously and said he had always been a teetotaller.

On examination he was a well-spoken, elderly man who looked older than his stated age. He was untidily dressed, with his shirt buttoned incorrectly. He was slow to reply to questions and he was lacking any facial expression. He was preoccupied with worries about his health and was concerned he might have cancer. Although he appeared depressed, he denied feeling so. He denied any suicidal thoughts and there were no psychotic features. Occasionally he forgot the question he had been asked and his concentration was impaired on clinical testing. He was very slow to answer tests of orientation, but was fully orientated.

Opinion

First episode depressive illness. Associated with psychomotor retardation and neglect. Requires further assessment of cognitive state and physical health.

Management

He was offered admission to a general adult psychiatric ward for further assessment of his mood and physical health. This he readily accepted.

In the ward there was a marked diurnal variation in his behaviour in that he was agitated and preoccupied with his health first thing in the morning, and gradually his mood and behaviour became more normal towards evening. Physical examination and investigation revealed no new physical illness. Although his concentration was obviously impaired, there was no other evidence of dementia. A diagnosis of depressive illness was confirmed and he was started on a course of antidepressant drug therapy.

Case history 3 — assessment and management: the chronic schizophrenic sent home

A 50-year-old man who lived in lodgings asked to see the duty psychiatrist at a hospital late one evening. He said 'It's the voices, doctor', and went on to describe auditory hallucinations telling him to jump in front of a car. He told the doctor that he had spent several years in hospital because of his illness before moving on to a hospital hostel before discharge to the community 1 year ago. He said he did not like his lodgings and did not get on with his landlady. He added that people in the lodging house were 'being horrible' to him. On further enquiry the doctor learned that he received an injection fortnightly from a community psychiatric nurse (CPN). The patient said the drugs were not working and requested admission. The doctor discovered that the patient's psychiatric notes were signed out to his CPN. A telephone call to the CPN revealed that, in fact, the patient had a very good landlady with whom he had an excellent relationship. Unfortunately she was about to retire and the patient would soon need new lodgings. The CPN told the doctor that the hallucinations were longstanding and that the patient had never attempted suicide. She felt his condition had been unchanged recently, but suggested that she visit him the next day.

Examination revealed an untidy, dishevelled man, whose trousers were held up by a brightly coloured neck tie. His speech was circumstantial and difficult to follow. He repeated himself a lot, particularly complaining about 'the voices'. He described hallucinations in the form of voices talking about him, and telling him to harm himself. There were no delusions and there was no cognitive impairment. He was physically well.

Opinion

Chronic schizophrenia. No evidence of relapse. Presentation precipitated by accommodation worries.

Management

The doctor told him that his CPN would visit the next day and reassured him that he was not deteriorating and did not require admission. Reluctantly, the patient left the hospital and went home.

The CPN visited the following morning, assessed the patient, confirmed his mental state was unchanged and told the patient that the social worker from the rehabilitation team would visit soon to discuss his accommodation with him.

Case history 4 — assessment and management: the patient with acute psychosis admitted

A 30-year-old married man was brought to a psychiatric hospital by his wife and his mother-in-law. He worked as a joiner and the family lived in a second floor flat. He came carrying a bag of children's comics.

He was seen together with his wife. He told the doctor that he had no problems and had 'never been better'. He felt his wife and mother-in-law were worrying unnecessarily and he wanted to go home. His wife reported that for the last week he had not been sleeping and had been up most of the night carrying out 'do-it-yourself' work on their flat. The previous night he had stayed up all night to tile the kitchen. Earlier that afternoon he had told her that he wanted to build a swimming pool under his bed. She caught him trying to saw a hole in the floor through to the downstairs flat in an effort to build the pool. He was unconcerned by the fact that there were neighbours below who might object to this and planned to flood the hole with water. He had told his wife that he was going to finance this project by selling his 'priceless antique commando comics'.

There was no relevant family history. He had no past psychiatric history and there was no history of drug abuse or alcohol abuse. He was physically well.

Examination revealed a restless, agitated man who paced around the room and was reluctant to sit down. He talked non-stop about his plans for the flat. The doctor was unable to elicit evidence of any hallucinations or delusions. The patient was expansive and socially inappropriate e.g. he offered to sell the doctor one of his 'priceless' comics.

Opinion

Manic illness. No obvious precipitants.

Management

It was explained to the patient that he was ill and that his mood was rather too good, unrealistically so. He was told that if this was not treated he may come to harm and that he needed admission to hospital. His family agreed to this but he refused. With his wife's consent the doctor detained the man using an emergency section of the Mental Health Act. With the help of his wife he agreed to go to one of the wards where he was prescribed 100 mg chlorpromazine orally up to 4-hourly on an as-required basis. He accepted medication that evening and had a more settled night's sleep.

Case history 5 — deliberate self-harm

A duty psychiatrist was called to a local casualty department. That afternoon a 48-year-old divorced ice-cream vendor had been brought to the department by his niece. She had called unexpectedly to his house and found him lying on a sofa, having taken an overdose of sleeping tablets. She had found a number of legal documents by his side and he had left two envelopes containing money and addressed to his two employees in his ice-cream business. He was interviewed about 4 hours after gastric lavage and he was fully alert.

He told the psychiatrist that he had been a stupid man doing what he had done. He explained that he had made a number of mistakes in the financial management of his business which meant he would have to lay off his two employees. He had divorced from his wife about 2 years ago and had moved then to the locality. He had few friends and spent most of his time working in an ice-cream van. His 20-year-old unmarried daughter had recently fallen pregnant which led him to believe he must be a failure both as a father and businessman. He explained that in a moment of weakness he had suddenly felt it was all too much for him and had impulsively taken the sleeping tablets prescribed for him 2 weeks ago by his GP. He had been sleeping poorly recently and sat up most of the night trying to make sense of his accounts. He denied any family history or past history of psychiatric illness. He was a non-smoker and said he rarely had time to take a drink.

On examination he was a smartly dressed, middle-aged man who sat with his head down, avoiding eye contact. Often he would shake his head and reproach himself about the mess he had made of his business and what an embarrassment this would be to his family. He spoke in a monotonous voice. He denied feeling depressed as such, and denied any further suicidal thoughts or plans, reproaching himself for his temporary weakness. There was no evidence of psychotic features. His concentration and orientation were normal.

With his consent, the psychiatrist telephoned his niece. She was most concerned about her uncle whom she thought had been worrying unnecessarily about his business in recent weeks. As far as she knew his business was thriving. She confirmed that he had been deeply upset by the news that his unmarried daughter was pregnant. On direct questioning, she revealed that the patient's brother had suffered a manic illness.

Opinion

Depressive illness. Presentation precipitated by deliberate self-harm of significant suicidal intent.

Management

It was explained to him that many of his concerns may be features of a depressive illness and he was offered admission. In the ward he expressed ideas of hopelessness, poverty and increasing pessimism about his future. These beliefs were associated with several biological features of depressive illness. When he once more admitted that he regretted he had not taken his life, he was started on a course of ECT to which he responded well.

Case history 6 — threat of self-harm

A 22-year-old unemployed man who lived in bed and breakfast accommodation presented himself to a casualty department late one evening. When seen by the casualty officer, he produced a beer bottle and threatened to smash the bottle and then cut his wrists. The duty psychiatrist was called while the man waited peaceably in a cubicle.

When the psychiatrist arrived, the patient complained that he felt so depressed he was going to have to kill himself. The psychiatrist explained that both he and the patient would have to be safe during the interview and persuaded the man to give up the beer bottle. The patient insistently repeated that he was depressed and that unless something was done he would kill himself. With some difficulty, the psychiatrist found out that the patient had recently been on holiday which he had enjoyed. He said that his depression had started on the previous day. The psychiatrist also eventually learned that the patient shared a room with a friend who that morning had given him money to place a bet on the horses. The patient had gone into town and spent the money instead on a haircut and some new clothes. He was now frightened about what his friend might do to him and said it would be impossible for him to return to his digs.

The patient denied any family history of psychiatric illness. He told the psychiatrist that he had previously been depressed and had required inpatient treatment when a teenager. He denied any other worries. He smoked cigarettes and occasionally cannabis. He had not had any drugs recently and earlier that day had consumed two pints of beer. On his way to the casualty department, the psychiatrist had checked at the local psychiatric hospital to see if there were psychiatric records for the patient. When he was 16 years old he had been seen by a child and adolescent psychiatrist because of truanting and solvent abuse. At that time his mother was trying to raise a large family on her own. He had also been seen at a different casualty department about a year before in very similar circumstances. On that occasion he had threatened to cut his throat with a razor but had been discharged. He had only ever harmed himself once when he was 16 years old when he had taken an overdose of painkilling tablets. There were no biological features of depressive illness. On examination his smart haircut and new clothes were apparent. He was animated and adamant in his talk. His manner was insistent and at times threatening. He did not appear depressed. He was not self-reproachful and there were no psychotic features. His concentration was not impaired and he was fully orientated.

Opinion

Relationship crisis leading to accommodation problem. No evidence of psychiatric illness.

Management

The psychiatrist sympathized with his distress, but explained that he
did not think that he was mentally ill. The patient reacted angrily and
demanded to know what the psychiatrist was going to do to help him.
The psychiatrist enquired of what friends or family he had locally and
with the patient's consent telephoned his elder brother who was
prepared to take him in for the night. He was discharged from the
casualty department without any psychiatric follow-up.

Case history 7 — unrecognized drug-induced psychosis

A 22-year-old single cocktail waitress was brought to a casualty
department by her girlfriend late one night. The friend explained to the
casualty officer that for the past 3 days the patient had been weeping
and was terrified that people were following her. That evening she had
been unable to go to bed and her friend had persuaded her to come to
the hospital. She had been unable to go to her work as a cocktail
waitress for the past 3 days. The psychiatrist called in at the local
psychiatric hospital on the way to the department. The patient was not
known to the psychiatric services. When the psychiatrist entered the
interview room, the patient burst into tears and explained that she saw
shadows and felt that people were following her. She could not describe
clearly what sort of people were following her, but she believed that
they were evil and intended her harm. This was always worse when she
went to bed, and that evening the shadows had been so frightening that
she had agreed to come to hospital. She was constantly terrified and
had been unable to remain on her own in her flat.

Her girlfriend explained to the psychiatrist that she was normally a
happy-go-lucky person who had changed suddenly 3 days ago. The
friend knew of no reason for the change. She said that occasionally she
and the patient would go out drinking at the weekend, but she denied
any alcohol or drug abuse. The psychiatrist did notice that the friend
was expensively and fashionably dressed, and quite matter of fact about
her friend's distress.

On examination the patient too was expensively turned out. Her
make-up was smeared because of her tears. She wept continuously and
was obviously terrified. Her talk was appropriate and coherent and
there was no evidence of thought disorder. She was not self-reproachful
and denied any suicidal ideas. She described what sounded like visual
illusions, but more clearly described persecutory delusions of reference.
She was fully orientated and her short-term memory was intact.

Opinion

First episode paranoid psychosis. Cause uncertain and admission for
assessment appropriate.

Management

Both the patient and friend accepted admission readily. On arrival at
the ward, the patient was immediately recognized by one of the night

nurses. The nurse revealed that the patient was a prostitute who spent large sums of money on amphetamine and cocaine. Two months before she had had an admission under similar circumstances, but using a different name.

Case history 8 — a violent patient

The duty doctor in a psychiatric hospital was called one evening to an admission ward to see a 25-year-old man with a psychotic illness, probably schizophrenic. It was the patient's first ever episode of illness which was characterized by persecutory delusions. He felt he was being followed by cars, and that neighbours and then other patients were talking about him. He also felt people were able to put thoughts into his head against his will and expressed the belief that 'my son has been taken from me'. That day he had been started on oral chlorpromazine in a dose of 200 mg b.d. He had refused his evening medication. During the evening he had become increasingly suspicious and withdrawn, remaining in his room. Two nurses had entered the room to attempt to persuade him to take his medication. He threw the medication over the nurses, smashed a chair and brandished a chair leg at them, telling them to stay away.

The nurses left the room, immediately contacted their nursing officer, and obtained assistance from two male nurses on a neighbouring ward. The doctor was called at this point. The patient refused to see him and threatened to hit him with the chair leg if he attempted to enter the room. With the consent of the patient's wife, the doctor detained the patient under an appropriate emergency order of the Mental Health Act. The doctor and four nurses entered the room whereupon the patient retreated into the far corner. The patient was told who everyone was and was told that staff believed that he was ill. The doctor explained that he was going to give him an injection which would make him feel better and make him less frightened. The patient swore and said he would not accept the injection. The explanations were repeated. The staff approached him together, one grabbed the chair leg and the others each held a limb. There was a brief struggle but no one was hurt. He was put in bed, face down and given 10 mg droperidol i.m. Two nurses remained to reassure him. He settled and 20 minutes later agreed to take oral medication. He was given the chlorpromazine dose he had missed earlier and his routine medicine was increased to 200 mg chlorpromazine t.d.s.

Case history 9 — a homeless ex-prisoner

A 22-year-old single man arrived late at night at an emergency psychiatric clinic. He had been released from prison that morning after a 30-day sentence for non-payment of fines relating to drunkenness offences. He had drunk several pints of beer that day, but did not appear drunk. He told the duty doctor he was depressed because he had nowhere to stay and had no money. He insisted he needed to be in hospital, saying 'my nerves are shot to pieces'.

He had no past psychiatric history. He had fallen out with his family who in any case lived some distance away. He had three previous convictions for theft and drink-related offences.

On examination he was clean and tidy. He did not appear anxious or depressed, and was matter of fact in his manner. There was no evidence of psychiatric illness, although he was persistent in his demands for admission.

Opinion

Homelessness in a newly released prisoner.

Management

The doctor explained to him that he was not mentally ill and hospital admission was unnecessary. The patient became angry and said 'So you're doing nothing then'. The doctor sympathized with his plight and told him he might be able to help him find accommodation for the night. A telephone call to the emergency social work service resulted in his being found overnight accommodation in a hostel for homeless men. The social worker also arranged for him to be seen the next day by a colleague who referred him to an association concerned with the rehabilitation of offenders (NACRO). The association helped him find accommodation with a landlady later that day and also arranged attendance at one of their day centres.

Case history 10 — post-traumatic stress disorder

A 30-year-old married man with two children was brought to a psychiatric hospital by a social worker. Earlier that day he had attended the social work department for advice on debts he had accumulated. In the course of his interview with the social worker he had said he felt that life was no longer worth living.

The doctor found out that 7 months before he had been the victim of a vicious assault. He owned a 'fast food' shop in a city centre. When he was locking up one evening, he was attacked from behind by four youths who covered his head with a sack. They dragged him back into the shop, kicking and punching him. He was hung upside down by the ankles and threatened with castration. They raided the till and before leaving, poured petrol on him and over his shop, threatening to light it. Fortunately, they were disturbed by passers-by and fled. Since the incident he had rarely been able to leave his house because of panic attacks when he went into the street. He had regular nightmares about the incident and found himself reliving it from day to day. He had never been able to return to his shop. In the last month he had become increasingly depressed with suicidal ideas. He spoke very little, even to his wife with whom he had not discussed the incident; he thought it was 'unmanly' to share his problems with her. He had lost his appetite and was unable to enjoy anything.

There was no past psychiatric history. His difficulties had been compounded by loss of income and his inability to pay off loans which he had taken on the basis of his previous high earnings.

On examination he was anxious and agitated, wringing his hands constantly. He looked downcast and talked self-reproachfully about his debts and his lack of 'manliness' in being unable to cope. Although he had had suicidal ideas, he was adamant he would not act on these for the sake of his wife and two children. He had no psychotic symptoms. Orientation was normal, although his concentration was impaired.

Opinion

Post-traumatic stress disorder complicated by depressive illness.

Management

It was explained to him that the stress he had experienced was out of the ordinary and that his difficulty in coping — far from being 'unmanly' — was both reasonable and understandable. He was reassured that he could be helped to cope with many of his symptoms, e.g. his low mood could be treated with antidepressants and his panic attacks treated by psychological methods. He was asked to return the next day with his wife. She confirmed the degree of his depression and his GP was advised to prescribe a sedative antidepressant. Follow-up was arranged in which his phobic symptoms were dealt with behaviourally — with his wife's assistance. During the follow-up he was enabled to speak to his wife about the incident and his subsequent experiences. He improved considerably, but it was a further year before he returned to work (not in his own shop which he sold). Even then there were some residual symptoms, e.g. occasional nightmares about the incident.

Case history 11 — undiagnosed physical illness presenting psychiatrically

A middle-aged Indian man was brought to a casualty department by the police. That evening he had been standing in the middle of a road, shouting and gesticulating at passers-by. While being interviewed by the police, he began clutching at the air as if to catch something. His speech was incoherent and he was unable to give any personal details. The police said they had seen him wandering in the streets over the past few days. He had been living the existence of a down-and-out and had obtained food by begging at Indian restaurants. The casualty officer who interviewed him suspected that he had experienced visual hallucinations and noted that he had been living the life of a down-and-out. He diagnosed delirium tremens and contacted the duty psychiatrist. He did not physically examine the patient.

Opinion

Delirium tremens in an immigrant of no fixed abode.

Management

The duty psychiatrist heard the provisional diagnosis over the telephone, and suggested that the patient be sent directly to the local psychiatric hospital. The patient was not seen by the duty psychiatrist. On arrival at the psychiatric hospital, the patient was clerked by the duty senior house officer. The patient was incoherent, unable to communicate but was visibly distressed. He was a small, coloured man of Indian appearance who was obviously underweight. He appeared to be dehydrated. His pulse was regular at 130 beats a minute and he was tachypnoeic. Auscultation of his chest revealed widespread rhonci and crepitations, particularly affecting the left upper zone. Shortly after admission he was incontinent of faeces. The duty senior house officer was so concerned about the patient's physical condition that he arranged immediate transfer to a local hospital specializing in diseases of the chest. Shortly after transfer, the patient died. A postmortem revealed that the cause of death was septicaemia secondary to pneumonia caused by *Klebsiella pneumoniae*.

Final diagnosis. Acute confusional state secondary to pneumonia.

Case history 12 — a visit to the police cells

A duty psychiatrist was asked to attend a police station where a 40-year-old labourer has just arrived. He had been arrested after a series of disturbances at his neighbour's house and in the street. When he arrived at the police station he began to express odd ideas, and did not permit anyone else to come into his cell. On his way to the police station, the duty psychiatrist visited the local psychiatric hospital to find the man had no psychiatric case records. The man lived with his wife and children. Normally he worked as a labourer but he had not gone to work that day. The police were called during the afternoon to a neighbour's house where the man had broken down the door, entered the house and thrown the television set from the window. He had then stolen a bronze statuette from the neighbour's house, gone out into the street and began to smash car windscreens with the statue. On arrival at the cells he had sought the corner of his cell and defied anyone to enter, threatening anyone who did with physical harm.

When the psychiatrist approached the cell door the man was pacing the cell. When the doctor introduced himself the man went to the corner of the cell and shouted that no one should come near him. The man was bare-chested, appeared to be extremely frightened and was sweating heavily. When the psychiatrist commented that the man looked frightened, he agreed and told him that this was the fault of other people who were talking about him and threatening him. At this he said no more and would not elaborate.

With the man's consent, the psychiatrist telephoned his wife. His wife informed the psychiatrist that her husband had been well until that morning when he did not go to work. He had appeared unusually irritable and started to mutter about the neighbours. It was shortly after that he left the house to break into the neighbour's house. On direct questioning his wife admitted that her husband was a heavy drinker, spending most of his pay on drink. She had to work to keep the house and look after the children. They had rowed a lot about this and 2 days before he had promised he would try to cut down his drinking. His wife knew of no other physical or mental illness.

Opinion

Working diagnosis of delirium tremens. Necessary to exclude other causes of paranoid psychosis.

Management

The man was too suspicious to agree to leave the cell and go to hospital. With the consent of his wife, he was detained under an emergency section of a Mental Health Act. The psychiatrist explained to him that his fears were the result of illness and that he would be taken to a local hospital. The police agreed to take him to the intensive care unit of the local psychiatric hospital. On arrival he was immediately prescribed 15 mg diazepam q.i.d. and given an i.m. injection of multi-vitamins. His psychosis resolved completely within 4 days.

Case history 13 — dementia — with social problems

An 85-year-old married woman was brought to a casualty department one morning by the police. They had been telephoned by a concerned neighbour who had seen the patient wandering in the street in a distressed state. The old lady had told the police that she was looking for her husband who hadn't returned from work. The police learned from the neighbour that her husband had been admitted to hospital the previous night because of a heart attack.

The duty psychiatrist was called to casualty. The old woman told him as she had told the police that her husband was at work in a local factory (he had retired 20 years ago). She was unable to give a reliable history and was disorientated in time and place (she didn't realize she was in a hospital). The psychiatrist telephoned the patient's GP who confirmed that the husband was in hospital and would be there for 1 or 2 weeks. The GP told the doctor that the patient had been increasingly forgetful over the previous year and relied heavily on her husband. He added that she had been physically well and was on no drug therapy. He knew that she had one daughter who lived several hundred miles away. On examination the woman was alert and fully conscious although disoriented in time and place. She was dressed in outdoor clothes but was wearing slippers. She was talkative and confabulated, e.g. she said she had just been to see her daughter that morning, which was impossible. She seemed unconcerned and was no longer distressed. There was no evidence of depressive illness or psychosis. She was unable to tell the psychiatrist the day, date or time. She was unable to recall any of an address 5 minutes after she had been given it. A physical examination was carried out and revealed an irregular pulse rate, 86. Her blood presure was 135/85. There were no other physical abnormalities of note.

Opinion

Dementia. Presentation precipitated because of withdrawal of normal social support.

Management

The two main needs were increased support to cover the period of her husband's hospitalization, and further assessment and investigation to establish the cause of her dementia. The psychiatrist telephoned a psychogeriatrician and was able to arrange assessment at a psychogeriatric day hospital the same morning. She was supported by an emergency day hospital placement on 3 days a week. The social worker in the psychogeriatric unit contacted the home care organizer and arranged home help on the remaining week-days until her husband was fit again. Further assessment and investigation was arranged through the day hospital.

Case history 14 — acute confusional state

A psychiatrist working in a general hospital was telephoned by a surgeon colleague with an urgent request that he see a 72-year-old man who had 'become psychotic'. The surgeon reported that the previous night the patient had refused a night sedative saying that the nurses were trying to poison him. During the night he had been restless and had got out of bed on several occasions. When he had been asked why he had got up he had told the nurses that there were intruders in the ward and that he had to deal with them. He said he had seen them at the end of his bed, adding that 'They were dressed up as policemen'. In the morning he was more composed and although no longer suspicious of the nurses, still felt that 'something funny' had been going on in the ward the previous night. Three days before the patient had undergone a transurethral resection of prostate. He had been well preoperatively and the operation had gone well with no complications. His only medication was nitrazepam 5 mg nocte which he had taken for years.

When the psychiatrist arrived in the ward, the nursing staff confirmed the details of the history. A look at the case notes revealed no important past medical history and no mention of any psychiatric history. Both the house officer and the nurses were clear that the man had been well until the previous night. The house officer reported that on his night round he had found the patient remonstrating with a drip stand which he thought was a neighbour who had come to harm him. When this misinterpretation was explained to him he had settled.

On examination the patient was then lying quietly in bed. He was disorientated and thought he was at home. During the interview he became drowsy on several occasions and had to be shaken by the psychiatrist to keep him awake. He could not recall refusing his medication the previous night and said he got on perfectly well with the nurses. When questioned, he said that there had been policemen in the ward during the night and that they had been summoned because patients at the end of the ward had been having a noisy party. He also revealed that in the last day or so he had heard voices calling his name. He would not cooperate with attempts to carry out cognitive testing, saying 'This is nonsense', and 'Why are you asking me this?'

Opinion

Acute confusional state. Repeat physical examination and investigations required to establish aetiology.

Management

Physical examination revealed signs of a chest infection which was confirmed by X-ray. Urea and electrolytes were normal. Blood gases revealed that he was hypoxic with a Po_2 of 9 kPa. The patient was told he had a chest infection and commenced on an antibiotic and oxygen via nasal cannulae. His sedative was stopped. The psychiatrist advised medical and nursing staff how to approach and manage the patient. In accordance with his suggestions, the patient was moved to the bed nearest the nursing station, the numbers of staff involved in his care were minimized. Staff were reminded to introduce themselves, constantly reorientate the man and explain everything they did to him. Although he was again disturbed that night (he thought someone was under his bed), he was successfully managed without sedation. His condition improved over the next 5 days.

Appendix 3
Specimen letters to GPs

First contact

Dr Strangelove,
The Surgery,
Bunkerhill,
Edinburgh.

Dear Dr Stangelove,

Re: Miss L. Muffet, Webb Street, Edinburgh — d.o.b. 10.12.50

Miss Muffet was brought to the Emergency Clinic on 21st
March 1989 by her sister, Mrs Cobb. She has had no previous
contact with the hospital.

Present problem. Mrs Cobb complained that Miss Muffet
drank excessively. Mrs Cobb lives in Glasgow and arrived in
Edinburgh today to find her sister intoxicated. Miss Muffet lives
alone in her own flat and holds down a good job as a sales
manageress in a local store. She told me she drank about a half
bottle of vodka each day and slightly more at the weekends. She
denied any medical, social or psychiatric problems because of
her drinking, and has not sought help for her drinking.

Examination. Miss Muffet was well turned out and spoke
coherently and appropriately. There were no features of
psychiatric illness or alcohol withdrawal, and she denied any
thoughts of self-harm. She, unlike her sister, was quite
unconcerned about her drinking.

Opinion. Heavy drinking. Referral precipitated by concern of
sister.

Management. Miss Muffet did not require any emergency
treatment today. I am not sure she would accept help for her

183

drinking, and I have not arranged any follow-up. I told Miss Muffet and her sister about local agencies that help with alcohol problems, and suggested they might discuss these options further with yourself.

Yours sincerely,

Dr Crippen
Psychiatric Registrar

Already in psychiatric treatment

Dr Strangelove,
The Surgery,
Bunkerhill,
Edinburgh.

Dear Dr Strangelove,

Re: Jack Horner, Victoria Street, Edinburgh — d.o.b. 01.04.38

Mr Horner was brought to the Emergency Clinic on 21st March 1989 by his daughter, Mrs Plumb. Mr Horner has suffered from schizophrenia for 20 years and attends fortnightly at the Continued Care Clinic to receive injections of fluphenazine decanoate.

Present problem. Mrs Plumb complained that the voices Mr Horner heard had been worse over the past week and that her family found it hard to cope with him. Mr Horner is a divorced man who normally lives with another daughter in Edinburgh. This daughter has recently separated from her husband and he has been staying with Mrs Plumb for the past week.

Examination. Mr Horner was untidily dressed but not neglected. His behaviour and speech were appropriate. He had a mild facial dyskinesia. He described auditory hallucinations of several voices holding conversations about him; occasionally he spoke back to them. He was unconcerned about these and he told me he had had these for many years. This was confirmed by his case records. There were no new psychotic features. He had no ideas of self-harm.

Opinion. Chronic schizophrenia. No evidence of relapse. Referral precipitated by family crisis.

Management. Mr Horner did not require additional psychiatric treatment. Instead I have offered increased support for the family. As I informed you over the telephone, a community psychiatric nurse will visit Mrs Plumb at home this afternoon. If her advice and support is insufficient, it may become appropriate to offer Mr Horner a respite bed in one of the hostels. This can be discussed further when he attends his routine appointment at the Continued Care Clinic on 25th March.

Yours sincerely

Dr Crippen
Psychiatric Registrar

Appendix 4
Psychotropic drug side-effects in emergency psychiatry

This appendix will cover only those psychotropic drug side-effects which require immediate management, or those side-effects which may be misdiagnosed as symptoms of psychiatric illness in emergency practice:

— Neuroleptic drugs:
   • Akathisia
   • Acute dystonia
   • Pseudo-Parkinsonism
   • Sudden confusion
   • Neuroleptic malignant syndrome
— Lithium toxicity.
— Adverse reactions to monoamine-oxidase inhibitors.

NEUROLEPTIC DRUGS

Neuroleptic drugs are used to treat psychoses, and the major classes are:

— Phenothiazines, e.g. chlorpromazine, thioridazine, trifluoperazine and depot preparations such as fluphenazine decanoate.
— Thioxanthenes, e.g. flupenthixol and clopenthixol.
— Butyrophenones, e.g. haloperidol and droperidol.
— Diphenylbutylpiperidines, e.g. pimozide and fluspirilene.

   In the early stages of treatment with any of these drugs the following syndromes may present suddenly:

Akathisia

— Distressing motor restlessness, often most marked in the lower limbs.

— May occur early or late in treatment.
— So unpleasant that it may lead to disturbed behaviour in an ill patient.
— Not to be confused with motor symptoms of psychosis (see Ch. 5).

Treatment

— Reduce dose if possible.
— Not treatable by anticholingergic drugs.
— No guaranteed pharmacological treatment.
— Oral, or if urgent, parenteral long-acting benzodiazepines, e.g. diazepam, may be helpful.

Acute dystonia

— Sudden involuntary contraction of muscles.
— Clenched jaw.
— Extrusion of tongue.
— Occulo-gyric crisis.
— Opisthotonos.
— Usually in younger patients.

Treatment

— Parenteral administration of anticholinergic drugs:
  • Procyclidine 5–10 mg i.m./i.v.
  • Orphenadrine 20–40 mg i.m.
— Reduce dose of offending drug if possible.
— Remember that neuroleptic drugs are long-acting and oral anticholinergic drugs may be required for days after neuroleptic treatment has been discontinued.

Pseudo-Parkinsonism

— Rigidity and akinesia, with tremor less apparent.
— Usually appears early in treatment but may occur at any stage.
— May be associated with hypersalivation.

Treatment

— Also responds to anticholinergic drugs but less likely that parenteral administration will be necessary.

— Initial oral dose:
  • Procyclidine 5 mg t.d.s.
  • Orphenadrine 50 mg t.d.s.
— Do not prescribe anticholinergic drugs routinely to cover
  neuroleptic-induced side-effects because:
  • Gut motility is altered
  • Metabolism of neuroleptic drugs is increased in the
    liver
  • May promote tardive dyskinesia
  • Euphoriant effects may lead to abuse

Sudden confusion (atropine psychosis)

Neuroleptic drugs like chlorpromazine and thioridazine have
strong anticholinergic properties. In susceptible patients, or in
high dose, or in combination with anticholinergic drugs,
atropine psychosis is an important cause of sudden
confusion:
— Visual hallucinations.
— Restlessness.
— Acute confusion.
— Signs of cholinergic blockade:
  • 'Red as a beet'
  • 'Dry as a bone'

Treatment

Neuroleptic and anticholinergic drug therapy should be stopped
immediately. Patients should be managed in accordance with the
guidelines for acute confusional states (see Ch. 13).

Neuroleptic malignant syndrome

— Hyperthermia, muscle rigidity and autonomic instability, e.g.
  fluctuating pulse and blood pressure.
— Usually associated with the most potent neuroleptic drugs,
  e.g. fluphenazine or haloperidol.
— Symptoms may appear days or weeks after treatment
  started.
— Exhaustion, dehydration and concomitant physical illness
  may be important aetiological factors.
— Mortality is significant and it may be up to 20%.

Treatment

— Stop neuroleptic drugs.
— Body temperature must be reduced.
— Dehydration must be treated if present.
— Detailed physical assessment is essential and any concomitant physical illness must be treated.
— Muscle tone may be reduced by dantrolene (10 mg per kg orally).
— Bromocriptine (60 mg per day orally) may enhance dopaminergic activity.

LITHIUM TOXICITY

Lithium toxicity is the result of excess (>1.5 mmol/l) of lithium carbonate in the blood. This may be precipitated by:

— Excess intake.
— Dehydration.
— Inhibition of lithium excretion in the kidney by drug interaction:
  • Thiazide diuretics
  • Non-steroidal anti-inflammatory drugs
  • Phenylbutazone
  • Tetracyclines

The symptoms of lithium toxicity increase in severity as serum concentration of lithium increases. Early symptoms are:

— Anorexia.
— Vomiting.
— Diarrhoea.
— Coarse tremor.
— Unsteadiness.
— Dysarthria.
— Sleepiness.

Late symptoms include:

— Impaired consciousness.
— Neurological abnormalities:
  • Fasciculation
  • Nystagmus
  • Hyperreflexia
— Convulsions.
— Coma.

— Death is likely when serum lithium concentration rises above 4 mmol/l.

Treatment

— Stop the intake of lithium carbonate.
— Serious toxicity is a medical emergency.
— Treatment is by saline and osmotic diuresis.
— The diagnosis may be confirmed by a blood test. Note the time of the last dose.

ADVERSE REACTIONS IN PATIENTS' TREATMENT BY MAOIs

After a spell of being out of fashion, monoamine-oxidase inhibitors (MAOIs) are once again commonly prescribed for certain phobic and depressive illnesses. Important adverse reactions in patients receiving these drugs may be precipitated by foodstuffs, or interactions with other drugs. The interactions with foodstuffs are usually only unpleasant, but the interactions with drugs are potentially fatal.

Reactions precipitated by foodstuffs

Foodstuffs containing monoamines such as tyramine and phenylethylamine are:

— Cheese.
— Degraded protein, e.g. pickled herring or pâté.
— Yeast and protein extracts.
— Alcoholic drinks.
— Vegetables, e.g. broad bean pods, green banana skins.

These may produce:

— Flushing.
— Pounding headache.
— Rise in blood pressure.
— Rarely the rise in blood pressure is severe.

Treatment

— Usually no treatment is required.
— If more severe, chlorpromazine 200 mg orally.

Drug interactions

Interactions of the MAOIs may be precipitated by:

— Sympathomimetics, e.g. amphetamine-like drugs, proprietary cold cures.
— Pethidine.
— Tricyclic antidepressants.
— Rarely any class of sedative drug, e.g. alcohol, phenothiazines.
— A mild syndrome similar to that with foodstuffs may be seen.
— More serious symptoms resembling overdose with MAOIs:
  • Agitation
  • Hallucinations
  • Hyperreflexia
  • Hyperpyrexia
  • Convulsions
  • Cerebrovascular accident

Treatment

— Stop all drugs.
— Cardiovascular signs may be treated as above.
— Severe reactions may require chlorpromazine 50 mg *slowly* i.v. or phentolamine 2–5 mg i.v.

Appendix 5
Advice for HIV-positive patients

GENERAL ADVICE

— Eat a healthy diet. (Avoid restrictive faddish diets.)
— Avoid food products containing raw eggs or non-pasteurized milk.
— Take regular exercise.
— If possible keep up regular interest, hobbies or work.
— Avoid excesses of alcohol, cigarettes or other drugs.

PRECAUTIONS AGAINST SPREAD OF INFECTION

— Preferably avoid vaginal and anal intercourse.
— Avoid unprotected intercourse. Always use a condom with a water-based lubricant, preferably containing the spermicide nonoxinol 9.
— Have safer sex, rather than simply less sex.
— Do not donate blood.
— Do not share a razor or toothbrush.
— Do not share a hypodermic needle.
— Blood or vomit should be cleared up with paper towels and flushed down the lavatory.
— Soap and hot water or dilute household bleach are sufficient to clean household surfaces once mopped by a towel.

PRECAUTIONS AGAINST INFECTION

— Promote kitchen and household hygiene.
— Follow defrosting and cooking instructions meticulously. Most foods will have to be cooked thoroughly.
— Do not store food outside the refrigerator and then reheat.
— Cuts or grazes should be kept clean and covered with a waterproof dressing.

— Any skin contamination should be washed immediately with hot soapy water.
— Avoid close contact with pets.
— Avoid having ears pierced, acupuncture, tatoos or being shaved in a barber's shop.

ADVICE FOR WOMEN

— Pregnant seropositive women are at a higher risk of developing full-blown AIDS.
— Most babies will also be seropositive.
— Most seropositive babies do not survive.
— Breast milk is a definite route of transmission of HIV.

SAFER SEX

— No body fluids such as semen, urine or blood should come into contact with mucosal surfaces or broken skin. Anal intercourse frequently causes small tears of the rectum.
— Safe sex techniques include: masturbation, kissing and massage.
— If intercourse cannot be avoided, follow guidelines above on condoms.
— Condoms must not be re-used.
— Take care that the condom does not slip off during intercourse.
— Hold on to the condom after intercourse to prevent leakage of semen.

THE GOOD NEWS

HIV cannot be spread by shaking hands, hugs, crockery, lavatory seats, towels or day-to-day contact with other people.

Index

Page numbers in **bold** type refer to Case Histories.

195